BREAKNECK BOOTY

THE 19 MOST EFFECTIVE, NO-EQUIPMENT EXERCISES
TO STRENGTHEN, GROW, AND TRANSFORM YOUR
GLUTES FROM HOME IN JUST 14 DAYS

SHELBY KENNEDY

CONTENTS

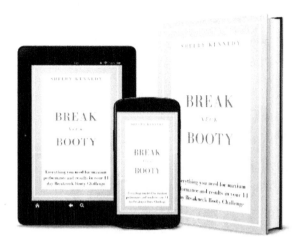

A Special Gift To Our Readers

Included with your purchase of this book is our Breakneck Booty Reference Guide. It gives great tips and advice to grow your glutes faster and get results!

Scan the QR code below to let us know what email to send it to:

For my husband. You make loving fun.

ABOUT THE AUTHOR

"The journey of a thousand miles begins with just one step..."

— LAO TZU

Shelby Kennedy is an entrepreneur and author born in the small town of Gibsons, British Columbia, Canada. She lived in Vancouver for 10 years before moving out to enjoy life in the more peaceful interior, where she now lives on her 42-acre spread with her childhood sweetheart, their daughter, four dogs, and two horses.

Shelby is the owner of two successful construction companies. She is also a fashion, lifestyle, and fitness content creator on Instagram. Now Shelby is embarking on a new course and adding another thread to her entrepreneurial skills. She is writing books aimed at providing women with workouts that leave them with a sense of accomplishment.

In her free time, Shelby enjoys fashion, working out, and spending time with her family. She loves food, experimenting with new recipes, and cooking something delicious for her family every night. Traveling is one of her greatest passions. Shelby took an eight-month solo trip spanning China, Australia, Indonesia, and Thailand, trekking through part of her journey on a motorcycle.

Shelby's main aims in her professional life are to help women feel good about themselves, enable them to become empowered, and provide them with the tools that allow them to take control of their health and body. Shelby wants the women who read her books to feel proud after completing their workouts. Shelby dreams of one day becoming a permanent resident of the Caribbean.

You can contact or follow Shelby Kennedy at

Instagram: @itstheshelblife
Email: shelby@breakneckbody.com

INTRODUCTION

I have a good friend named Kim. She's now in her mid-30's, settling into a sedentary lifestyle and working a nine-to-five office job. She gets up at 7 a.m., wakes up her kids, gets them dressed and fed, and walks out the door by 8:00 to drop the little ones off at daycare on her way into work.

The highway into the city is always packed in the morning, but it's worse when she's leaving work in the evening. She gets stuck in traffic way longer than she wants. Once she picks up her kids, she rushes home to make dinner and get them in bed. Kim wakes up and does it all again the next day.

Kim loves her family and her job, but she doesn't have a whole lot of 'me-time.' She looks at her to-do list every day; it is always overflowing with work deadlines, soccer practices, social events, and countless errands. Her wellbeing never makes it onto the list. She's so busy looking after her family that she can't fit in time to work out and look after herself. Kim wakes up in the morning exhausted and over-whelmed; it's so much easier to just stay in bed a little longer and catch those last few Z's until she needs to get up and start her day.

Kim is getting frustrated with this lifestyle. She often finds herself looking in the mirror and remembering her body before her children. She kept a few of her favorite pieces of clothing from back then with the goal of one day wearing them again.

She thought about going to the gym but being around all those gym buffs made her feel uncomfortable and self-conscious. She tried diet plans, but they became boring and repetitive. Besides, who wants to make two different meals for dinner every day? What's the point in cooking one meal for herself and another for everyone else?

I have another friend named Ashley. Ashley is a hard-working career woman in her late 20's. She has a high-up managerial position in a successful business where everyone needs something from her at all points of the day. She works tirelessly at the office, but her work often carries over into her home life. She burns out quickly by the end of the day.

Ashley promises herself that she will find the time to head to the gym later, but she always finds herself too tired or too swamped by the end of her workday. She goes home feeling disappointed and critical of herself. She spends most of what little time she has on the weekends catching up with friends or relaxing. She scrolls through Instagram and longingly looks at posts by fitness trainers and wellness coaches. Ashley wishes she could look like them. She actively reads their advice captions, watches their workout routines, and knows what she needs to do, yet the cycle continues.

Does this sound familiar? Do you know Kim and Ashley? Maybe you are Kim or Ashley. There's no shame in that—we're all busy women trying to have it all. We're all doing our best to achieve our goals and afford our dream vacations. We want our families to be happy as we try to balance our social lives; we want to work hard and make money to afford a house or a nice car. Sometimes our own health and fitness get put on the back burner until we have more time or energy.

We all do it! It's not something to beat yourself up over. It's something to acknowledge and address. Sometimes life gets in the way, and sometimes work and family take precedence over our own health and fitness.

You're not lazy. You're not a lesser woman than the Yoga moms who workout in the park every Tuesday or those Instagram influencers who do CrossFit livestreams every morning at 6:00 a.m. (that's a superpower, I swear). You are an individual living your best life and trying to make everything work. I applaud you for that—you're doing a great job!

But sometimes, you need a helping hand to guide you toward your personal goals.

Let's talk about you for a second. Who are you?

You're a hardworking woman living your best life and trying your hardest to make everything work. You're a family person, you're social, and you enjoy life. But something still feels missing.

Maybe you're a student working your way through college with a steady stream of classes to attend and overdue assignments piling up. You're staying up until midnight most days to finish those last few details. Then you're up at the crack of dawn, grabbing a coffee and running back to school to do it all again. Your fitness and health take a backseat to your grades and social life.

Maybe you're single and ready to mingle, but you feel uncomfortable in your own body. Going out with your friends feels like a chore. No matter what you wear, you never feel confident in how you appear.

We women are constantly being judged for our bodies. We eat a big burger and overhear whispers that we eat too much; we eat a salad and get asked if we're eating enough. Our weights constantly fluctuate, when we're on our period, when we eat a big meal, after childbirth, or as we age. Whenever we get bloated and go up a dress size, people ask us what's wrong or comment that we're letting ourselves go. Every time we wear loose clothing or go down a dress size, people start to ask if we're ill. We can never seem to look right for other people, can we? Then we look in the mirror and wonder how we can fix it all.

Here's your reminder: you don't need to fix anything about yourself. You are perfect just the way you are. Your body is a beautiful vessel; thank it! Seriously, go look at yourself in the mirror right now and thank your body. That's the first step in your journey of creating a happier and healthier body.

Unfortunately, exercise and food only get you so far. You need to remind yourself that your body is a wonderful, incredible part of you every chance you get. I challenge you to look in the mirror every morning and say to yourself, "I am beautiful. Thank you, body, for helping me achieve my goals every single day. Thank you for allowing me to do the work I need to do while looking after my family and friends."

The number one thing you need to take away from this journey is self-love. Once you can love yourself as you are, you are that much closer to reaching your wellness and fitness goals. You deserve more confidence, a positive outlook, a happier sense of self, and the healthier day-to-day lifestyle you are trying to find!

Welcome to your 14-Day Breakneck Booty Challenge! Over the next two weeks, our goal is to help instill that confidence in you once again by teaching you quick routines and exercises that you can easily knock out in your precious spare time. Your time is your choice. Your fitness is your choice. Let's help you learn how to make that choice and run with it!

In this book, we'll explore different exercises you can do in a short span of two weeks. These exercises will help you achieve a stronger, more toned body. You will also learn how to couple your exercise regimen with a positive outlook of yourself in order to create a well-rounded body, mind, and soul. You deserve to be as happy and healthy as you possibly can be, and that involves both your inner and outer beauty.

Let's push ourselves to be better, little by little. Our bodies are capable of incredible things. The next two weeks will prove that to you! A healthy lifestyle is not just about losing weight and being skinny or following the latest fad diet. Maintaining a healthy lifestyle is about learning to love yourself again.

I'm a confidence-first, fitness-loving lady. I do everything I do for my own motivation and to motivate others to be just a little better than how they feel right now. I've been training my body and learning to love it my whole adult life. I've been teaching women that their bodies are limitless. You can have it all, and you deserve it all.

I want women to realize that their full potential is already inside them. You can eat the foods you love, spend time with your family and friends, advance in your career, and still have time for yourself. Workouts don't need to take up all your time to be effective. It's time to enjoy life and let your fitness grow with you.

Over the years, I've learned that we are all on our own journey. Our lives are all their own paths, twisting and guiding us. Our paths are crossing for a brief moment as you read this text, and I hope you can take a little wisdom, advice, and confidence with you on to the rest of your journey.

Over the next 14 days, we'll be exploring short exercises you can incorporate into your everyday life to help you achieve your dream body and be more confident. Let's dive in and smash these next 14 days like the strong, powerful women we are!

1

NO GYM? NO PROBLEM!

It seems like the fantasy of the "perfect body" is everywhere these days—we can't escape it. Every time you open social media, there's another weight-loss hack or another device to sculpt your abs—for only four easy payments of $19.99!

Of course, we all want to achieve our ideal body! Whether or not we realize it, we're always on a path to bettering ourselves. But is our dream body as achievable as these influencers claim? Will all our stress and problems disappear? Will we be able to juggle our homelife and social lives, meet all our deadlines, and still look our very best while doing so?

All these things seem like they were created for people who have countless hours a day to spare, money to burn on supplements, and endless heaps of motivation. It makes the myth of an achievable perfect body seem inaccessible and almost impossible for you to achieve!

But a better version of yourself is not entirely beyond your reach. There isn't a quick fix or life hack to make you healthier, stronger, or fitter overnight. However, there are more sustainable and accessible ways for the average, busy woman such as yourself to reach your goals.

Your fitness journey doesn't need to be strenuously filled with hours upon hours spent at the gym, and it doesn't need to be thousands upon thousands of dollars spent on equipment. It doesn't need to take away from your family time and your commitments. It especially doesn't need to consume your whole life.

Your fitness journey is specific to you. You can mold it into whatever you want and need it to be at any particular time.

COMMON CHALLENGES

Everyone faces challenges on their fitness journey—you are not alone! But all the most common challenges have simple solutions. You never need to feel like your fitness dreams are incompatible with your lifestyle. Let's look at some common challenges or roadblocks you may be facing as you begin your 14-Day Breakneck Booty Challenge!

Not Having Enough Time

No matter what your daily life looks like—whether you're married or single, with or without kids—it always seems like we're too busy for 'me-time.' It can feel impossible to fit exercise into your day.

Women especially struggle to fit in time for fitness when our culture and society expect us to look after others and drop everything to help. There are plenty of expectations on our shoulders. We can sometimes put ourselves and our own needs on the backburner.

I want you to step back right now and ask yourself, how much time do you spend on self-care each day? I don't mean just face masks and Netflix. Do you notice that when you try to prioritize yourself, you are immediately busy with other things for other people?

It's true that we don't always know where the days and hours go. We get up in the morning, and a second later, it's lunchtime. One minute after that, you're getting everyone ready for bed. The next thing you know, everyone is all tucked in while you clean up from the day to prepare for whatever mess will happen tomorrow.

You must become aware of both your daily activities and the energy you exude on them. This can help you find time in your schedule to focus on yourself! Try keeping an hour-by-hour diary of your day for at least a week. This way, you can see what free time you have and keep track of it.

Once you find that free time, be sure to use it for yourself, doing things you enjoy and know will benefit you, like physical activity! Using your free time wisely doesn't mean you need to spend all of it working out. Forcing yourself to engage in physical activity at every opportunity throughout the day would be very unrealistic. You want something sustainable that can help you recover from your busy schedule and focus on yourself. Spend a bit of your free time working out; 20-45 minutes is a great start. Once you are done with your workout, you can spend the rest of your free time relaxing.

If you split up your free time between fitness and relaxing, you can give your muscles a chance to burn then rest. Taking that time to work out then rest will allow you to focus your mind on something other than the stressors in your life for a bit. You deserve it.

On your 14-Day Breakneck Booty Challenge, we've created daily workouts that span between 10 to 20 minutes of your day. As you begin, you may find yourself needing more breaks, which could increase your time. Remember—this is your time. It's okay to take the necessary breaks.

As the days go on and your reps increase, you'll notice the workouts will get longer and longer. Your first day may only take you about 10 minutes, whereas your last day may take you 30. As you build up your stamina, the increased time will mean you're improving your fitness each day and proving your strength.

It may be best to schedule 30 minutes each day to tackle these workouts. By planning and setting aside that time, you can ensure you have proper rest time the first few days and enough time in the latter days to complete your entire workout.

Finding Exercise Boring

The truth is that not everyone is meant to be a fitness guru or an Instagram model. Not everyone loves going to the gym for three hours a day, lifting the same weights over and over again, or running in place on a treadmill. And that's okay! Your fitness needs to be yours completely—as long as your fitness regimen fits your lifestyle and serves you, then you are on the right path.

Everyone has their own personal exercise preferences. Not everyone likes the same workouts, and not every workout will be beneficial or enjoyable for every person! You've got to figure out what works for you.

Once you figure out what works for you, you can roll with that. Your fitness should be fun and engaging for you. When your workout is enjoyable, you're more inclined to complete it and feel better afterward.

That being said, once you find the fitness routine you enjoy and that serves you best, you've got to remember to switch it up. Many people believe that you must do the exact same workout every day to make progress, but that simply isn't the case. In fact, the opposite holds true: you want to target your different muscle groups each day to keep working them out and build your strength. Changing up your exercise routine helps promote more muscle gain and weight loss by challenging your body to not stay stagnant.

How can you make your workouts more engaging? Shaking things up helps, but you can also add some extra external influences. Try playing a podcast or putting on a TV show. Find something you enjoy paying attention to when your side starts cramping up or when you think of stopping. Distracting yourself like this encourages you to keep going! Focusing on something else takes a bit of your focus and helps take your mind off the burn or the nagging thoughts to do something different! Refocusing is another way to stay engaged.

Avoid growing bored from exercise by exploring different types of fitness, switching up your workout every once and a while, and finding some external stimuli to help keep you distracted as you exercise.

Feeling Like You Aren't Doing Enough

We can get caught up on social media and forget that it isn't real life. Instagram can make you compare yourself to others and feel like everyone else is better off than you or is doing better than you. Comparing yourself can make you think you have to spend hours every day at the gym to see results. If they can be a working mom who runs around from place to place and spends a handful of hours in the gym each day, then why can't you?

That nagging thought isn't true.

Research indicates that you don't need to follow such a strict fitness regime to see results. The amount of time you work out is only one factor that goes into your fitness. Four main factors go into your fitness: the frequency, intensity, duration, and type of exercise. These factors work together to help you achieve your fitness goals.

The American College of Sports Medicine (ACSM) recommends that adults spend about 30 minutes five days a week participating in moderate-intensity aerobics or 20 minutes three days a week participating in vigorous activities to see results (Sprow, 2019).

It's funny how 20 minutes a day three days a week doesn't seem like a lot, does it? That amount seems like a more manageable number, but it still adds up to a whole hour of exercise! If it can be as effective as what those fitness influencers achieve in all those hours, then what's the harm? Anyone can make time for 20 minutes every other day.

Or does it still seem like a lot of time for you? Luckily for you, the ACSM also states that any physical activities at least ten minutes long also see benefits. This finding means that even if you're only able to work out for ten minutes, you're still making progress! A little progress every day is much more beneficial than none at all.

As you start incorporating fitness into your daily routine (or alternating days routine), you'll notice how much easier it is to work out more. Sooner or later, you'll find that 20 minutes is no problem. Then 30 minutes comes easy; then 40 minutes! It may take you time to build up to those amounts, but it is actually pretty easy to whip out a 40-minute workout when you've worked up to it and feel good about it.

The key to increasing your workout durations is to lay out a plan before heading into your workout. Know what you're going to do each day; that way, you can immediately jump in, rather than wondering what to do next. You can research different exercises to target the specific muscles you want to target, then plan accordingly. You can follow trainers' videos on social media or video-sharing platforms! You can even join challenges you see online or via workout apps, which can guide you along your journey, providing you with dedicated exercises and regimens to help increase your stamina, strength, and workout time! This 14-day plan is an excellent example of that—a regiment you can follow to help improve your duration and create your best breakneck booty!

Not Enough Energy to Exercise?

We're all feeling very overwhelmed and stressed these days. Everyone is always busy running around between work and social events, balancing spending time with family and friends. Feeling tired or rundown is understandable. You're not alone feeling like your exhaustion is endless.

It may feel counterintuitive, but when you exercise and exert energy for fitness, you actually encourage more oxygen and nutrients to flow through your body to your muscle tissues. Doing so will improve your health and provide you with more energy (Mayo Clinic, 2019). Isn't that so strange? You'd think that moving your body so much would exhaust you more, but that is not the case! In fact, a little physical activity each day can help you produce a chemical called adenosine triphosphate, which provides you with more energy to tackle your day.

The U.S. Department of Health and Human Services suggests that the average adult needs about two and a half hours of physical activity a week to experience the full benefits of exercise (Webb, 2011). If you partake in the 20 minutes for every other day as suggested, you're already well on your way to meeting their suggestions. More energy reaches your muscle tissues, producing more adenosine triphosphate, the primary energy source for most cells. All of the rewards you reap culminate in progress on your way to reaching your goals. It's simply proof that a little bit of movement and exercise a day is better than nothing at all.

At first, you may have a hard time finding the energy to start moving. However, within just a short time period, you'll be reaping the rewards that come with more physical activity in your life. Find ways to motivate yourself when you are starting out by setting rewards for yourself after your workout. I like to reward myself with a healthy, protein-filled snack and some family time. Find what works for you. Encourage yourself to start moving, and the energy will come more naturally.

Tried in the Past and Failed

One of the biggest obstacles women face, is getting discouraged after trying and failing to reach their fitness goals. This discouragement is worsened by the influx of Instagram influencers praising all sorts of exercise fads and the benefits of hours in the gym. It can be challenging to find motivation when you try repeatedly without achieving the same results as them.

The most important thing is to not give up. Try re-evaluating where things went wrong, what you want to get out of your workouts, and then manage your expectations from there. Were you trying to do too much in each session? Did you set unrealistic goals for yourself? Were you not challenging yourself enough? Were you focusing on Instagram instead of on your own enjoyment and energy?

Think about where you went wrong and figure out how to continue in a healthier, more accessible manner. Remember that you need to pace yourself and set realistic goals. If you decide to try working out thirty minutes five days a week, then set that goal and follow through on it. You'll start to see results over time without overwhelming yourself!

If the goal you set proves to be too much for you, don't stop altogether! If you are trying to work out too frequently, reduce your workouts from five days to three. After consistently maintaining your revised goal, slowly add to it over time to build it back up again.

Trust your body to tell you what it wants and needs. You're capable of more than you realize. Even if you aren't able to reach a particular goal at this point in your journey, that doesn't mean you never will be able to. You can reduce the duration of your workouts to increase your stamina, you can explore other types of movements, or you can return to the basic fundamentals of exercise. Taking the time to go back to basics can help you reach your goals in a healthier manner.

In short, your fitness goals are achievable. There are always going to be roadblocks along the way. Some days, you may feel like you'll never reach those goals. Do not give up! You're capable of a lot more than you think. Your fitness journey is yours to explore and enjoy. It's all a part of your self-care routine.

You may hit roadblocks, like getting bored when working out or not knowing how to continue through sore muscles. However, you should know that there are easy fixes to overcome these challenges. Try a variety of different solutions, like finding workout buddies to help push you through the bad days or playing a podcast in the background to distract yourself. You can try a combination of stretching and taking a soak in a nice, hot bath to relax your muscles. There are so many ways to solve these problems. Don't let the little things stop you from reaching your goals.

The Breakneck Body Squad is a Facebook group for everyone embarking on this same fitness journey as you. It is a great place to go if you ever need encouragement. Our group is also a place where everyone can ask questions about exercise without fear. It's a great reminder that we're all on this journey to self-improvement and creating a great body and a breakneck booty together!

Each person on their fitness journey experiences ups and downs. The Breakneck Body Squad's Facebook group is all about providing a supportive community for women to share their journeys and support one another. In this community, we share our progress, wins, favorite exercises, videos, form and posture tips, and even recipes! It is a positive, encouraging, and safe space to share, track, ask questions, motivate, and make connections with other women on their fitness adventures. I urge you to like, interact with, and support each other in the group. I am always available inside the Breakneck Body Squad community to ensure your further success! You've got this!

2

THE GLUTES, EXPLAINED

Since we are focusing on toning our booties, you may find yourself wondering, what exactly is your gluteus maximus? You've heard fitness instructors always talk about how great your booty looks when you work those glutes, but what exact muscle groups are you working out? Which muscles should you be targeting? After all, your glutes are more than just your booty. Understanding your whole body and the muscles you're trying to target will help you find the best exercises for your specific goals.

THE FOUR MAIN ASPECTS OF YOUR BOOTY

In layman's terms, the gluteus maximus is a collection of the three muscles in your booty area. But your gluteus maximus muscles aren't the only aspect of your butt! Four parts of your body contribute to making and shaping your butt: your bone structure, your subcutaneous fat, your skin, and your muscles.

Bone Structure

Your primary bone structure in the booty area is the pelvis. Your pelvis is the part of your skeletal system that forms the shape of your hips and creates the structure of your butt. You may often hear trainers talk about tucking the pelvis or building flexibility in your joints to support your pelvis. It's a major player in the balance of your lower body, especially when doing exercises in Tabletop Pose (on all fours with a flat back, tucking in your chin).

Subcutaneous Fat

The subcutaneous fat layer covers the majority of our bodies. Many people believe that you want to burn away as much fat as possible to form a better-looking booty, but there are places where it's healthy to keep a layer of fat. Your booty needs subcutaneous fat for protection when you sit and to make your day-to-day activities more comfortable. Other parts of your body that need layers of fat include your calves, back, and chest. Pre- and post-natal women especially need extra layers of subcutaneous fat.

Everybody has fat in their bodies. Fat is so natural, but everyone's fat distribution is different. Your fat distribution depends on your hormone levels and genetics. Despite the common myth, "spot reducing" isn't possible. Spot reducing means targeting specific areas of fat to minimize. When you burn fat, it burns from your entire body based on your genetics. I may workout and first notice the fat reduction in my arms, whereas you might do the same exercise and first notice less fat in your legs.

Despite wherever you visibly see weight loss, your body is burning fat off from all over. However, it is our genes that determine where and how we burn fat. When you really want to burn that extra fat around your booty, remember that you're actually toning that area while burning all the fat across your whole body. Burning your whole body's fat is a good thing! It means that your entire body is receiving the incredible benefits of exercise even though you're only targeting specific muscles. We target certain muscles to tone them, but we work out so that our whole body can lose weight and reap the benefits.

Skin

We can be very self-conscious of our skin, especially when we think of it as flawed. The skin on our booty goes through a whole lot; after all, it protects our glutes, which protect our pelvis. Our subcutaneous fat lies directly below our skin, which means that our skin can seem saggy if we haven't worked our glutes a lot.

We may also notice stretch marks spanning across our skin. Stretch marks are a normal part of life and nothing you should feel ashamed about. You are a strong and fierce tigress, and you should wear your stripes with pride. Stretch marks show how we've grown and changed, and every woman has earned her stripes.

The skin around your booty tends to work with your subcutaneous fat, helping with blood flow. Your skin is what protects your glutes from everything outside your body. You must look after the skin on your rear end. Ensure that you shower and scrub right after your workouts to clean off all your sweat and prevent unsightly pimples from forming. Opt for looser clothing to let your skin breathe, especially if you know you'll be sweating.

It's important to remember to take care of your skin and help its elasticity by moisturizing. If that works for you, do it! Everyone experiences dry skin, stretch marks, and acne in places we wouldn't expect. It's all normal. Just be sure to look after your skin, and it will look after you. Enjoy comfort and cleanliness to ensure the best results in your workouts!

Muscles

There are three muscles in your glutes: the gluteus maximus, the gluteus medius, and the gluteus minimus. These are the muscles you're going to learn how to target and strengthen. They help round our backside and provide padding when we sit. Our glutes help us balance, run, and walk! Each of these muscles has a specific job in the body, so breaking down what they do individually shows where all our hard work goes.

The Gluteus Maximus

The gluteus maximus is one of the largest muscles in your body, spanning from the base of your spine to the back of your legs in a spot known as the posterior gluteal line. The size of the gluteus maximus means it needs to be one of the strongest muscles in your body. It needs to support your lower body in your everyday activities like climbing the stairs, lifting, and lowering, as well as supporting your femur, thigh bone, and sacrum. Your gluteus maximus also serves you well in a lot of backward-kicking motions and exercises. You'll see this come into play when doing exercises like Donkey Kicks or Leg Lifts.

Most booty exercises target the gluteus maximus; they need to! Since the gluteus maximus is such a large muscle, it needs to be worked more to establish a better baseline strength. It's such an important muscle to ensure you're able to keep you with your day-to-day routines.

The Benefits of Strong Gluteus Maximus Muscles

Strong glutes help you in your daily activities by preventing muscular imbalances and overcompensation on other muscles. This just means, if your glutes are underdeveloped, other muscles in your body will have to help do the work. Oftentimes, your abs or leg muscles can become involved. Incorrectly using these muscles could lead to muscle strain and fatigue. Strained or fatigued muscles can really slow you down from running all of your errands or from accomplishing your goals. Hurting your muscles could halt your progress and put you back a few days.

Your gluteus maximus also supports your lower back. Strengthening your gluteus maximus helps relieve any lower back pain you may have. Keeping your glutes active will help reverse any stress on your back that a sedentary lifestyle causes.

As a bonus, stronger muscles tend to appear more prominently. Working your gluteus maximus will lead to not only better stabilization and movement but to a rounder and perkier-looking booty!

The Gluteus Medius

The gluteus medius, also known as the upper glutes, is a deeper layer of muscle that lies beneath your gluteus maximus. It is responsible for hip abduction and rotation. Your gluteus medius comes into play during sideways activities like Leg Swings or Side-Leg Raises. The upper glutes are also activated through the lateral rotation of your thigh towards the outside of your body, which you do during activation exercises like Clamshells.

Training the gluteus medius will help balance your booty's shape by rounding out its appearance. Your upper glutes are second-in-command for building that perky booty.

The Gluteus Minimus

The gluteus minimus is the smallest of the three gluteal muscles. The gluteus minimus is located even deeper than the gluteus medius, and it sits right beneath your upper glutes. The gluteus minimus is shaped like a fan, works with the gluteus medius in hip abduction, and helps support your pelvis when you walk.

Strengthening your gluteus minimus can help with hip joint stability, reduce your lower back pain, reduce any hip pain, and help improve your performance in other exercises, like running.

Your posterior has many other small muscles that are not necessarily trainable and do not lend to training, but they will be worked in turn as you work the bigger glute muscles. What does this mean for you? As you work and engage your major glute muscles, you will work these smaller muscles too. The gluteus minimus comprises your piriformis, your obturator externus and internus, your quadratus femoris, and your superior and inferior gemellus (Jolie, 2015).

LET'S GET GOING!

So much of your body goes into building a perkier booty. The same applies to every part of your body: to develop one area better, you need to develop everything else. Your entire body works together as one whole. Learning how the different parts of your body work together is key to creating the right workout routine for your goals.

In this 14-day challenge, I've put together different exercises specifically chosen for the groups of muscles and joints they target. As much as we're focusing on your booty, we're also going to be working out your abs, arms, and legs. Your whole body is getting a massive workout, which will add to the work we put into your backside. We're going to make you strengthen all of your muscles while focusing on that derriere extraordinaire.

I encourage you to do your own research into the other muscle groups throughout your body. That way, you can find different ways to incorporate other muscles into your workouts, especially through your abs. A strong core is your saving grace in terms of balance and forming a solid base for everything you do. Once you've established a base under-standing of all your muscles and how they affect every exer-cise you do, you can find the best workouts to suit your goals and needs.

Let's start here with this curated 14-day workout. I've done the heavy lifting for you so that you can learn to do the heavy lifting. We're going to build a perkier, breakneck booty together. As a bonus, we'll strengthen the rest of your body in the background as we focus on that butt. Let's be proud of the work we do. Now that you know the muscles in your lower body, you can begin your journey to the best and healthiest version of yourself.

3

DON'T SKIP THE STRETCHES

The most important part of your exercise regimen is your stretching. It can help at the beginning of your workout by getting the blood flowing and waking up your muscles, and it can help at the end of your training by soothing and loosening any tight muscles and beginning the recovery process. Stretching in between your workouts also helps relieve pain and increase your average daily flexibility! All these benefits will help you prevent injury when you exercise.

It's entirely way too easy to create tight glute muscles from sitting for long periods, especially when working a sedentary job or staring at a computer all day. In contrast, overworking your glutes has the same effect; they can also get tight from overexertion during workouts. No matter the cause, tight glute muscles will lead to discomfort or injury if not addressed.

A lot of our daily discomfort comes from having tight glutes and a tight lower back. You can relieve this discomfort and pain when you learn to release the tension and stretch out your muscles in these problem areas. Stretching your behind is beneficial to your glutes, your lower back, and different muscle groups all over your body. Stretching the glutes also helps you release tension and tightness in your hips, hamstrings, and even some of the pain you may be feeling in your pelvis and knees. That's right! Stretching one part of your body will help release tension in other parts of your body. Your whole-body benefits from doing these stretches.

Stretching your glutes also helps to enhance your flexibility, improve your range of motion, reduce your risk of injury, and improve your overall mobility. These attributes will help you later in life by preventing unnecessary surgeries and helping you retain mobility and self-sufficiency as you age.

It's best to stretch your glutes before and after your work-outs. There are benefits to both, so be sure to incorporate proper stretching into every workout. Doing so will make your workouts more enjoyable and prevent injuries.

10 STRETCHES TO RELIEVE TENSION IN YOUR GLUTES

You can use many different stretches to help relieve tension in your glutes and improve your overall mobility and flexibility. We will cover 10 various stretches for your glutes, but these are only a few of the many beneficial stretches available. Feel free to practice other stretches if some of these don't work for you. The stretches provided below are a great jumping-off point, but they are only the tip of the iceberg when it comes to stretching and looking after your booty and lower body.

Chair Glute Stretch

Another name for this stretch is the Seated Pigeon or the Seated Figure Four. As the name suggests, the Chair Glute Stretch is done in a chair. You can even do this exercise while sitting at your desk. If the chair proves to be too difficult or uncomfortable for you, you can also sit on the floor to execute this stretch.

Sit upright in your seat and place your right ankle over the left thigh, just above your left knee. Place your hands gently on your shins. From your seated, upright position, you should slowly and slightly lean forward to deepen your stretch. Hold this position for up to 30 seconds before slowly returning to the starting position. Be sure to repeat the stretch with your left leg on top.

The Chair Glute Stretch opens up your hips, but it also releases the tension throughout the outer leg and the side of your booty. You should be able to feel a good stretch through each side of your body, and you should feel more open through your hips afterward.

Be wary of how much you lean forward when executing this stretch. If your hips and backside are super tight, you may feel a bit of pain during your stretch. Don't push yourself further than you're capable of going. If the stretch begins to hurt or feel uncomfortable, try leaning a little less.

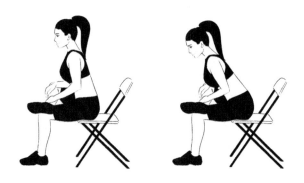

Seated Glute Stretch

The Seated Glute Stretch is very similar to the Chair Glute Stretch, but this one is set up on the floor. You want to sit similarly as before, with your back straight and your legs stretched out in front of you. If you feel any pain in your hips or lower back, make sure you sit on a yoga block or a folded towel. A softer, padded surface will help alleviate some of the pressure on your joints and bigger muscles.

To execute this stretch, lift one leg and place that ankle just above the other leg's knee. If you can already feel a great stretch in this position, then that's fantastic! Hold it there for up to 30 seconds. If you want a deeper stretch, begin slowly leaning forward and keeping your back straight; hold for up to 30 seconds, and then slowly bring yourself back upright. Don't forget to switch sides. Again, be wary of how far you lean. If you feel any pain, pull it back a bit. You don't want to strain your muscles or cause any more tension.

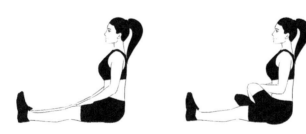

Downward Facing Dog

Downward Facing Dog is a fantastic traditional Yoga pose that aids multiple muscle groups, including your hamstrings, calves, shoulders, and glutes. Downward Dog is an incredibly versatile stretch. Keep this one in your repertoire no matter which part of your body you want to stretch.

Start in a push-up or Plank Pose with your hands directly under your shoulders and your legs together behind you. You must keep your back straight in this position and stay as flat and even as you can. Staying flat means do not dip your hips down towards the floor or stick your booty up, which creates a curve in your lower back. Both of these mistakes can be detrimental to your form and harm your body.

From the push-up position, move your hips upwards and backward to create the look of an upside-down V with your whole body. Slightly bend your knees and let your head hang down, your eye line looking back towards your toes, thus continuing the straight line you established in your Plank Pose. In this position, your eyes will be looking down towards the ground and your toes. Be sure to push your heels towards the floor to really feel the full benefits of this stretch.

You might not be able to get your feet completely flat, and that's okay! It takes a lot of practice to achieve a full Downward Facing Dog, so don't force anything your body isn't able to do just yet. Simply stretch your heels down as far as they'll go until you can feel the stretch through the back of your legs and hamstrings. In this position, you should also feel your shoulder muscles engage as you slightly pull your body away from your hands. If this stretch hurts or impacts your wrists at all, place a yoga block or towel beneath each hand.

Hold Downward Facing Dog for up to 30 seconds, then slowly roll your body back to the push-up or plank position. Afterward, repeat the entire stretch, moving slowly as you transition in and out of it. Ensure that your posture is correct. Since so much of your body is involved, make sure that you look after your whole body as you move. Listen to your body, and don't push it beyond its capability.

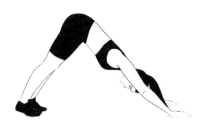

Pigeon Stretch

The Pigeon Stretch is another foundational Yoga pose that is great at grounding you. It helps release tension throughout your hips, back, and glutes. Execute this stretch correctly by starting on all fours, also known as Tabletop Pose. When you are in Tabletop Pose, remember to keep your arms and legs straight at a 90-degree angle from your torso. Your wrists should be directly below your shoulders, and your knees should be directly under your hips. Be sure to look directly down at the ground to retain a straight line from the top of your head all the way to your tailbone.

Let's imagine that we are starting on our right side. From the Tabletop Pose, lift your knees slightly off the ground, focus your energy on your shoulders rather than your wrists, and then float your right knee forward. Bring your right ankle to the opposite wrist. Your right leg will bend forward, across your body, with your knee and your shin facing away from you. Next, gently bring your right leg down to the ground as you slide your left leg back. Make sure the top of your left leg is touching the floor with your toes pointed behind you. Afterward, slowly lower your upper body over your right leg and hold.

Once in the holding position, walk your hands out ahead of you and stretch your arms forward, similar to your arm position in Child's Pose. Try to rest your forehead gently on the floor in front of you. If that proves to be too deep of a stretch for you, don't sweat it! Lowering yourself all the way to the ground is a more advanced technique. You may be able to master it over time, but don't hurt yourself by pushing yourself too far at first. Instead, keep your hands or forearms under your shoulders, and you can lower your upper body as deep as is comfortable for you.

Hold the Pigeon Stretch for the length of at least five deep breaths. A deep breath consists of a long inhale through your nose, feeling your belly expand, and a long exhale through your mouth, feeling your belly deflate. Alternatively, holding the stretch for up to 30 seconds while steadily breathing works too. After you finish, slowly bring your body back to the starting Tabletop Pose. As always, be sure to repeat the stretch by alternating it on the other side.

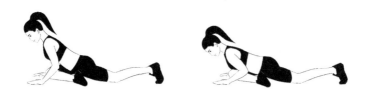

Knee to Opposite Shoulder Stretch

The Knee to Opposite Shoulder Stretch is excellent for anyone who suffers from sciatica pain; it helps loosen all the tension around your sciatic nerve. You may be familiar with this stretch if you've ever been to a chiropractor or physical therapy. Either way, the Knee to Opposite Shoulder Stretch is great for relieving any pain you may feel and is beneficial to your overall body health.

Begin by lying flat on your back with your legs stretched out beneath you, in line with your hips. Your arms should be down at your sides. Bend your knee and lift it towards your chest. Next, wrap your hands around the shin below your knee and slowly pull that knee up towards your opposite shoulder. Be very careful that you don't pull your knee too far away from your hip so as not to hurt yourself. Keep your hips glued to the floor beneath you for the entirety of this stretch.

Hold this stretch for 30 seconds before you return your leg to the ground. Don't forget to repeat this stretch on the other side. As always, be aware of how your body feels as you execute this stretch. Never push yourself further than your body will allow. If you feel any sort of pain, simply reduce your range of motion; there's no shame whatsoever in listening to your body!

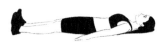 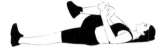

Seated Twist

The Seated Twist begins in a seated position on the ground, with your legs out in front of you and your toes facing upwards. To stretch out your right side, turn slightly and place your left arm behind your left shoulder. Next, bring your left leg up and over the right, placing your left foot on the floor near your right knee. Put your right arm around the bent left leg, letting your right hand's palm face away from your body. Slowly twist your upper body in the same direction as your palm, letting your arm gently pull the bent knee inwards.

Hold this stretch for up to 30 seconds before slowly unwinding. Make sure you alternate and repeat the stretch for your other side. When you perform this stretch, please be extra careful to keep your shoulders pulled down and away from your ears so that you don't strain your neck or carry extra tension. Double-check that your spine is as straight as possible to avoid added pressure on your lower back, spine, and pelvis. Imagine a string running up from your backside, through your spine, and upwards through the top of your head, pulling your body up and free. Picturing the string helps ensure that your back is as straight as possible and helps relieve some of that lower-body pressure.

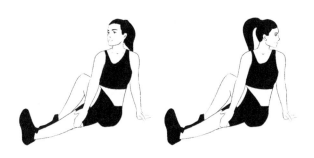

Lateral Hip Stretch

The Lateral Hip Stretch is great for releasing tension in your lower back and opening up your glutes and hips. This stretch is particularly great after a long day spent sitting at a desk in front of your computer.

To execute this stretch correctly, lie on your back with your legs bent so that your knees face upwards and your feet are flat on the floor beneath you. Keep your hips square and balanced.

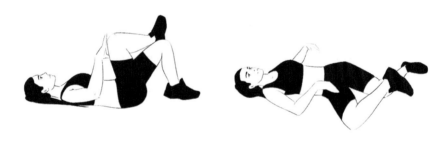

Starting with our right side again, place your right ankle over the left knee. Slowly lower your knees towards the right side. Remember to keep your back flat on the floor as you twist. Your lower back will naturally want to lift, but ensure that your upper body stays firmly pressed onto the ground beneath you. Push your arms toward the ground as you twist, and engage your abs to ensure your body stays in proper form to retain proper form.

Child's Pose

Child's Pose is another important stretch that is a Yoga building block. It works to open up your shoulders, upper back, and hips while stretching out your abs, low back, and glutes. Child's Pose is a wonderful way to thank your body for all it does for you. Some yogis also like to use this stretch to thank the Earth for holding them up.

Child's Pose also starts in Tabletop Pose. However, this time you will make sure your knees are out slightly wider than your hips. From here, slowly sit back onto your heels, letting your body lower between your legs. Stretch your arms away from you, resting your palms on the ground.

Keep your body still for as long as you can. If you're comfortable with it, try pressing your forehead down to the ground beneath you. Try holding this pose for up to two minutes, breathing in through your nose and out through your mouth. Afterward, slowly pull yourself back up to return to Tabletop Pose.

Keep Child's Pose in your back pocket as a quick tension release at any point in the day. This stretch is sure to become a favorite! Child's Pose is a quick way to engage with yourself and with the world around you; it grounds and calms you as it helps stretch you out.

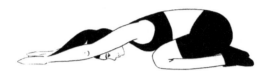

Yogi's Squat Pose

Yogi's Squat Pose can be a little tricky, but people love it once they get the hang of it. This stretch is fantastic for opening up your hips, energizing your lower body, and getting your blood flowing.

Start by standing with your feet slightly wider than hip-distance apart and your toes facing out a bit at the two and ten o'clock positions. Slowly bend your knees and squat down, keeping your back straight and your knees in line with your toes. In this squat, you want to go down as deep as you can while keeping your heels on the floor. It may take you a few tries to get all the way down without lifting your heels, and that's okay! This stretch will help you open up your hips as well as help lengthen your Achilles tendons and your hamstrings. Working on these areas will help you out big-time as you progress in this stretch and as you continue to work on opening up your lower body.

Once you've reached the full extent of your squat for today, go ahead and bring your hands together in front of you as if you were praying, keeping your elbows out to the sides. If you can, place your elbows between your knees for stability and to get a slight extra stretch through your inner hips.

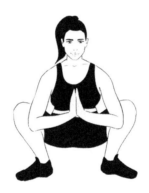

You can hold this pose for up to 30 seconds before bringing yourself back up to a standing position. Feel free to repeat as needed. Be sure to shake out afterward. If your Achilles tendons aren't used to being stressed like this, please give them a rest after performing this exercise. Don't push your body beyond its current capability. The more you practice and workout, the further you will be able to go with each pose.

Kneeling Lunge Stretch

The Kneeling Lunge Stretch is a personal favorite of mine. This stretch does wonders for your hips by opening them and releasing tension throughout your glutes and hamstrings. Start in a kneeling lunge. We will once again imagine that we are starting on our right side. Kneel on your right knee, with your right shin and ankle straight out behind you. You should have your left foot planted in front of you, with that foot lined up at a 90-degree angle directly under your knee.

Once you are aligned and in the correct starting position, place your hands on your hips and gently push your hips in front of you, down towards your knee. Remember to keep your core tight and your back as straight as you can. Hold this stretch for several slow, deep breaths. Be sure to breathe in through your nose and out through your mouth. After you finish holding the stretch, return upright, switch sides, and repeat the movement.

Be careful with how far you push yourself forward. You want to stay engaged and challenge your body without risking losing your form or popping your hips out of alignment. Keep your hips square and ensure that your forward knee does not go over your toes; this will help keep your form correct and avoid injury or strain. For that extra stretch, you can pull your back foot towards your bum, which stretches the thigh through the knee.

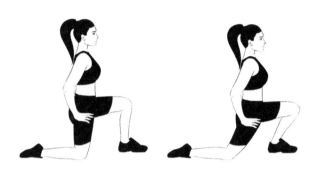

YOU GOT THIS!

Now that you've learned all your stretches, you're ready for the next step in your workout! Be sure that you begin and end every single workout with a few stretches. Your body deserves a little love, and stretches are a great way to give it just that. Stretching is a simple and easy way to keep your body flexible, get your blood moving, and increase mobility during daily activities.

Think about how much stretching could benefit you while playing with your kids or your pet! Think of how much pressure you could relieve from your back while you're at work or on your daily commutes! It will be so much easier to go about your day if you just spend a few minutes stretching.

You're on your way to achieving your dream strength and fitness goals. All it took was five minutes of stretches to open you up and get you started! Now nothing is stopping you from a few more minutes of exercise to show your body some love. Let's kick these next 14 days in the butt!

4

ACTIVATION EXERCISES

Most of us live relatively sedentary lifestyles. We spend a fair amount of time sitting at home, at work, or in our car. After being so inactive for hours on end, you need to prime your body before you jump into any of the resistance exercises we'll be covering. Activation exercises help you make the most of your workout and avoid injury. When your muscles haven't been working or are weak from inactivity, they need an opportunity to wake up and remember how exercise and engaging movement feels. If you don't give your muscles the chance to prepare, then at best, you risk less than satisfactory results; at worst, you risk injuring yourself or straining your muscles.

Certified Strength and Conditioning Specialist (CSCS) Holly Perkins states that activating your muscles before your workout helps form a connection between your brain, nerves, and muscles. Creating this connection helps better prepare your whole body for a successful, active, and engaging workout. Perkins shares that doing your activation series ensures "every rep of your strength-training routine [is] effective, even during the first set...Alternatively, if you begin your workout [without activating], your first set becomes your warm-up, and, in essence, a waste (Osnato 2020)."

There's another vital caveat regarding activation: if you've been working your booty a lot in your workouts and aren't seeing the results you want, activating your muscles could help you achieve those goals. Activation exercises can open your body up, get your blood flowing, get your muscles working, and wake up your glutes. Activation exercises guarantee these benefits no matter which muscles you're working. Doing so will ensure your muscles are working at their peak levels when you actually begin your workout, thus increasing your visual results. Exercise is not all about aesthetics and looks, but it's always nice to see evidence that all your hard work produces results.

Below are detailed descriptions of a few activation exercises I'd like you to try. Give each of them a go and find which feels best for your body. Explore which activation exercises make your muscles feel the most awake and aware. Take note of which exercises engage the most muscle groups. In your daily workouts, I've assigned you two activation exercises to begin each daily exercise routine. Throughout the 14 days, we'll alternate through these activation exercises so that you can experiment and find out which ones are the best for you. That way, you can learn to execute these activation exercises to your very best ability for optimal results.

DONKEY KICK

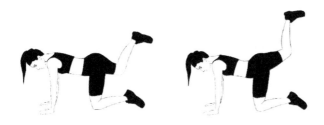

The Donkey Kick exercise, which mimics the look of the animal, targets your whole gluteus maximus. The Donkey Kick activates a large chunk of your booty and the deeper muscles below it.

Get onto your hands and knees in the Tabletop Pose previously discussed in the stretching section. Remember to check your form when starting with Tabletop Pose by slightly tucking your chin in towards your chest. Make sure that you keep your abs engaged to keep your back flat and your hips square. Engaging your abs also ensures that you maintain stability as you transition from one leg to the other.

Start with your right side. Retain the 90-degree angle you have in your bent legs as you raise your right leg towards the ceiling, the underside of your foot facing up to the sky. Squeeze and engage your butt muscles as you do so—don't forget to keep your pelvis tucked and your core engaged—then return your knee to the ground right before your back starts to arch. When you do this exercise correctly, you will look like a donkey kicking upwards. Repeat this motion on your right side to complete your right-side reps, then switch to your left side to complete the remaining repetitions.

Form Tips

Move slowly the first time you do this exercise. Listen to your body to help you identify when is a good time to return to your starting position after pushing your leg up to the ceiling. How far you push and how long you hold depends on your strength and flexibility, but you can learn a lot by paying attention to what your body is telling you.

Engaging your abs in this exercise will help you avoid arching your back and keep your lower back muscles from doing all the work. Keeping your form like this will instead make your glutes get to work. Engaging your abs also helps keep your hips level, which might be difficult if you have tight hip flexors or a tight iliotibial band. If you find this move difficult, try practicing it in front of a mirror at first. Either way, always be sure to lift your leg only as high as your hips can stay level.

Benefits

Once you find your perfect Donkey Kick form, you will reap the benefits of this activation exercise. Due to the level of stability this exercise requires, you will find that you work your shoulders and your core as well as your gluteus maximus. This exercise is great for toning those muscles as well. The Donkey Kick particularly benefits people who sit a desk job because it stretches your hip in the opposite direction of how it rests when you sit.

CLAMSHELLS

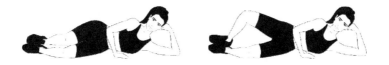

Clamshells target your gluteus maximus as well as your gluteus medius, so it's a very well-rounded move and will help wake up all the muscles in your booty and prepare you for your workout.

Let's imagine we're beginning our Clamshells on the right side. Start by lying on your right side with your feet and hips stacked. Rest your head on your left hand to hold you up, and put your right hand on your hip for stability. Bend your knees at a 90-degree angle. Keep your ankles lined up with your hips, and keep your knees facing out. Raise your right knee as far as you can without rotating your hips. As you raise your knee, keep your left leg on the floor and your feet pressed together. As always, remember to engage your abs and your core.

Hold this for a second or a beat, squeezing your glutes at the top, then slowly lower your knee back down to your starting position. When you do this activation exercise right, your legs should kind of mimic the look of a clamshell opening and closing; think about protecting that pearl inside. When you finish with your reps on this side, be sure to flip over and do the remaining reps on your left side by lifting your left knee.

Form Tips

Clamshells can be challenging to execute correctly and can easily lead to injury, so pay close attention to your form. Be sure to keep your neck in a neutral position when you do this exercise to avoid neck strain; keep your bottom arm under your head to accomplish this task. Tucking your bottom arm provides stability to your neck as you move your legs, but it also helps you think about this exercise as coming from your hips rather than your lower back. Focusing on your hip's movement properly isolates and engages your glutes rather than using your back muscles. For added stability, engage your core throughout the entirety of the workout.

Benefits

Once you've found the proper form, you can reap the benefits of the exercise. These benefits include strengthening your hips and decreasing your risk of a lower-body injury. Clamshells also help you build up your stabilization and balance, increasing the strength and power throughout your core and lower body. Clamshells are often used in physical therapy because they help ease and release your back tension, which helps with any back pain you may have. Clamshells target your gluteus medius, so it helps target your inner and outer legs while it strengthens your pelvic area. This exercise has a plethora of benefits!

DIRTY DOG (OR FIRE HYDRANT)

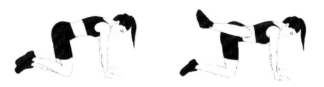

The Dirty Dog (also known as the Fire Hydrant) is another aptly named exercise. You can probably guess what it's going to look like just from the title. The Dirty Dog also targets your gluteus maximus and is very similar to Donkey Kicks.

The Dirty Dog is a very well-rounded exercise. It targets all areas of your hip mobility and glute functions. These functions are your extension, your internal and external rotation, and your hip abduction.

Hip abduction is the movement your hips and legs make off of your torso. These movements aid in day-to-day activities like getting in and out of your car. Your internal and external hip rotations also assist in basic, everyday activities like walking and running. Hip extensions are simply any movement that lengthens the front of our hips. We see this daily as we stand from a seated position. Our hips are ball joints, meaning movement in all different directions is possible, so it's essential to strengthen our hip muscles and joints in every direction and mode possible.

Start with the Tabletop Pose again. Don't forget to keep your back straight and neutral, align your wrists under your shoulders, and line up your knees under your hips. Make sure that you're looking down at the ground directly below you to retain a straight, flat back.

Start with your right leg first. Tuck your pelvis and engage your core to retain stability as you lift your right leg away from your center at a 45-degree angle. Think of your leg as a swinging door. Make sure you keep your knee bent at a 90-degree angle. Tuck the pelvis and engage your core to retain stability. Make sure your hips stay square and lined up with your shoulders as you squeeze your glutes at the top of this movement. When you are done, slowly lower your right leg back to the ground. Repeat this exercise until you've completed all your reps for your right side before switching to the left side.

Form Tips

Make sure you're staying safe and rotating your hip correctly. You can achieve this by thinking about pointing your toes to the wall you're lifting towards. Double-check that you are engaging your core and hips throughout this exercise for added stability. Ensure that your hips are the only parts of your body that are doing the actual moving.

Benefits

Once you perfect your form, the Dirty Dog sculpts your glutes and improves your posture. This exercise also helps to improve back pain when correctly executed. The Dirty Dog encourages stability by engaging your glutes and your ab muscles, enabling you to maintain a neutral spine.

The Dirty Dog benefits both your hip rotators and abductors through the extension of your hips and through the rotation needed to execute extending correctly. Working your hip muscles and joints helps you during everyday activities like walking, climbing the stairs, and dancing.

5

14 DAYS TO A BREAKNECK BOOTY: WEEK 1

W elcome to the first week of your 14-Day Breakneck Booty Challenge! Now that you have the basics down, it's time to dive right in!

During this first week, you'll be completing varying repetitions of each move every day. You will begin with 12 reps on day one and gradually increase to 20 reps by days six and seven. Pay attention to the changes in reps as the days progress. You don't want to overexert your muscles and exhaust yourself in the first few days, so please adhere to the suggested amounts of repetitions.

Take a one- to two-minute break between exercises as you see fit. However, you should keep these rest periods short so that your heart rate remains elevated, and your muscles stay engaged throughout your workout. If you can't take a shorter rest between moves, then that's okay, too! The important thing is to make sure you are properly resting your muscles to avoid straining them while still moving enough to keep your muscles engaged and your heart working.

Before you begin every workout, always make sure that you take five to ten minutes to stretch your muscles. Refer back to Chapter 3 and pick a few of the stretches that you liked the most. Try to pick the stretches you think help open up your hips and wake up your lower body the best. How your body reacts to these same stretches changes over time, which means that the stretches you pick should be personalized to you by the moment. Feel free to pick-and-choose stretches to switch up your warm-up routine each day. There are no set rules on which stretches are the best for you on any given day—it all depends on you! Listen to your body to figure out which muscles are the tightest and need to be stretched out the most for that day.

Following your brief stretching warm-up, the rest of your workout will consist of two activation exercises and three main exercises. Don't forget how important activation exercises are to get those muscles ready and to get your heart pumping. As we go along, do not hesitate to go back and review the techniques and tips for each of the activation exercises we covered in Chapter 4. There is no harm or shame in refreshing your memory to stay safe and avoid injury. That's the wonderful thing about learning your exercise routines from a book—it will always be here for you to refer back to if you get lost!

Are you ready? Let's go!

WEEK 1 EXERCISES

Let's start by breaking down each exercise that you are going to be doing this week. Let's make sure you know how to execute the movements correctly and without injury. Don't be afraid to re-read each of the descriptions and practice in front of a mirror before starting your full workout.

Throughout the first week, we will perfect the Glute Bridge, Straight Side Lifts, the Straight Leg Hold, the Single Leg Glute Bridge, the Outer Thigh Lift, Side Plank Hip Dips, and Squat Pulses.

Glute Bridge

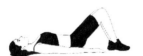 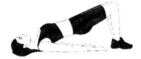

The Glute Bridge targets many of your larger muscle groups, guaranteeing that you will get a great burn. This exercise targets your abs, hamstrings, and gluteus maximus.

Instructions

Properly execute the Glute Bridge by lying down with your back on the floor. Place your arms by your side with your palms down. Keep your knees bent and your feet shoulder-width apart. Once your stance is correct, lift your hips off the ground while keeping your abs engaged. Your knees, hips, and shoulders should form a straight line. Once your hips reach the top of your movement, squeeze your glutes to really work them out. Hold that squeeze for a few seconds, and then lower your hips back to your starting position.

Practice proper breathing techniques. Be sure that you exhale as you raise and squeeze and inhale as you lower back down to the ground. Keep your breathing consistent as you continue through your reps. Consistent breathing will help engage the correct muscles and keep you focused.

Form Tips

Glute Bridges can be tricky to master, so pay attention to how your body feels. If you find that your hamstrings feel tight, try to move your feet a little closer to your glutes. The issue could be that you've simply stepped too far out of your range, thus targeting the wrong muscles.

If you start to feel the muscles in your back working more than your glutes, you may want to return to the starting position. Once there, reposition your back so that your hips are tucked and your abs are engaged. It's crucial to keep the majority of the work off your back to avoid injury. It's perfectly normal and natural to feel your back muscles doing a little bit of the work but be wary of how much you feel it. If your back muscles feel strained, painful, or obviously over-worked, then you should immediately stop, retreat to the starting position, and re-evaluate.

Maintain a neutral core and spine throughout the process. If you ensure that your core is engaged, the work should stay targeted where you want it. You can double-check that you activated your core by swaying your hips back and forth at the top of the bridge. If your core is engaged, you should be able to maintain your balance.

Straight Side Lifts

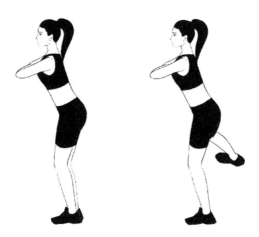

Straight Side Lifts are an excellent exercise for your gluteus medius and minimus, as well as your hips and thighs. This exercise actively works against a sedentary lifestyle by opening up your hips and waking up your lower body muscles. Straight Side Lifts also enhance your range of motion through your hips and improve stabilization.

Instructions

I prefer to do my Straight Side Lifts in a standing position to maximize the benefits, but some instructors will direct you to do this exercise from a sideways, lying position. Stand tall on your right leg without arching your back, holding your hands out in front of you for balance. Slowly inhale as you lift your left leg out to the side with your foot flexed. Do this movement as far as you can go without arching your back or bending to the side. You should feel a stretch in the top part of your booty where your hips meet your pelvis. Squeeze your glutes as you lift, especially once you reach the top of your movement; from there, exhale as you slowly bring your leg back down. Repeat and complete your repetitions on this side before moving to the left side.

You can hold on to a chair or wall for balance if necessary. The more you do this exercise, the more you can build up to just relying on your core for stability. Try to really contract sour abs and keep your eyes on one spot directly ahead of you to practice your balance.

Form Tips

During Straight Side Lifts, it is essential to make sure your hips stay aligned. If your hips push forward or back, you could be thrown off balance and strain your back muscles. Pay attention to your torso by letting your legs and glutes do the majority of the work. You want your torso to stay straight while making sure that your knees aren't locked.

Remember to always stay in control of your movement. Don't rely on momentum; rather, follow through by relying on the power and control of your muscles. Swinging and forcing should never be involved in any of the work you do. Keep your muscles engaged and use them to lift and lower yourself as you move slowly through each step.

Straight Leg Hold

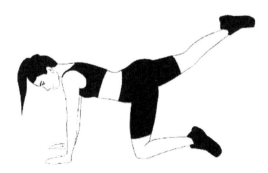

The Straight Leg Hold targets all the smaller muscles in your butt, like the gluteus medius and gluteus minimus. Targeting these muscles amplifies your booty work when you pair it with exercises targeting the gluteus maximus. It also targets your core, so you know this exercise is going to be a good one!

Instructions

Start this exercise in Tabletop Pose with your knees bent beneath you at a 90-degree angle. Keep your knees directly underneath your hips, and fully extend your arms. Keep your back straight and your eyes directly down, not looking behind you or ahead of you. You want to avoid looking around as it can and will cause neck and back strain.

From this position, raise one leg towards the ceiling until you feel your glutes begin to engage. Keep your leg straight with your foot flexed and the sole flat towards the ceiling. The important thing to remember here is that you should not be pointing your toes. Hold your legs in this position, keeping your muscles engaged and tense.

You should feel the muscles in your booty at the top of your movement. If you aren't feeling your muscles engaging, try reaching your leg a little higher up. If you do lift higher, be sure you aren't compromising your form just to reach higher. Don't forget to practice controlled breathing.

Form Tips

Be sure to keep your back flat and neutral the whole time. You mustn't curve your spine in this exercise to retain proper form and to avoid injury in your back. If you're not sure whether you're moving your spine, practice in front of a mirror or take a video of yourself to double-check your posture.

Single Leg Glute Bridge

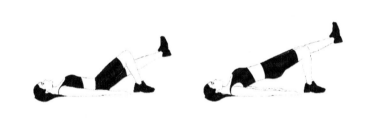

The Single Leg Glute Bridge is a hybrid that combines the Straight Leg Hold and the Glute Bridge, so it's one of the more advanced and evolved exercises. The Single Leg Glute Bridge challenges your balance while targeting all your glutes, hamstrings, and hip flexors. As you improve on this exercise, you may even notice some of your abs working too! Because of how many different muscles it incorporates, the Single Leg Glute Bridge is often recommended for athletes. This exercise is in beast mode!

Instructions

Start by lying down flat on your back with your palms facing down by your sides. Bend your knees and plant your feet shoulder-width apart. Be prepared to move into the exercise by making sure you are already engaging your abs and glutes.

Slightly tuck your pelvis by pulling your belly button towards your spine and then down your ribcage. Engage your core and lift your left leg off the ground, extending it straight. Be sure you're keeping your right leg bent and planted.

As you hold your left leg up, squeeze your glute and push your right foot into the ground. Keep your pelvis raised and level. Hold this position and squeeze your glutes extra hard for that final push. From there, lower your hips to your starting position. Repeat this movement on the other leg.

Form Tips

Remember to keep your chin tucked as you execute this exercise. Both of your knees should stay in alignment as well. Lastly, don't allow your back to arch; doing so may result in injury.

Outer Thigh Lift

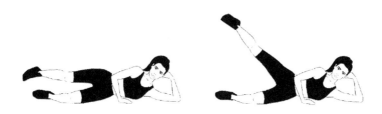

The Outer Thigh Lift is a versatile exercise that works your abductors and all three of the major gluteal muscles. This exercise is suitable for those interested in gymnastics, dancing, and even kickboxing. The added plus is that Outer Thigh Lifts also help with flexibility and toning your legs!

Instructions

Lie on your right side with your legs straight beneath you and your body in a straight line. Your hips, knees, and ankles should be in line with your feet. Keep your spine and neck straight so as to avoid injury. Bend your right elbow and rest your head on that bottom arm. Rather than placing your left hand on your hip, place that top arm on the ground in front of you. This placement helps rotate your pelvis forward slightly and isolates those glutes when lifting.

Exhale and raise your left leg, lifting it straight as high as you can without losing form. Keep your hips stacked. Your aim is to get your leg to at least a 45-degree angle (or higher) to get the most out of the motion. When you reach the top of the movement, squeeze your glutes before inhaling and lowering your leg back down to the starting position. After you finish the correct number of reps, alternate the exercise on the other side.

Form Tips

You must pay attention to your lines in this exercise. Keep your spine and legs straight throughout to avoid strain in your muscles. If your left hip rolls forward or backward, try lifting your leg a little lower. You may be extending your leg too high, thus causing tension in your hips or causing you to lose your balance and form.

Side Plank Hip Dips

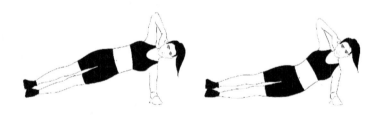

Side Plank Hip Dips are a variation on the classic Plank Pose. If you are familiar with Plank exercises, you already know that this will require lots of balance and core strength. This exercise targets each of the three major gluteal muscles and your obliques, also known as your side abs. Side Plank Hip Dips are a full-body move if ever there was one.

Instructions

To start this exercise, get into a Side Plank Pose. Lie on your side and prop yourself up on your bottom forearm, stacking your elbow directly under your shoulder. Your feet should also be stacked and in a straight line from your neck to your ankles. You can place your top hand on your hip or raise it towards the ceiling. Lift up your bottom side, pulling your hips away from the ground. If this feels too advanced for you, that's alright! Beginners can simply lower their bottom knee to the ground and execute this exercise in the Half Plank Pose. The important thing is that you progress at a pace with which you feel comfortable.

Keeping your body in a straight line and your chest open, drop your hips to the ground and lift right back up into the Plank Pose. Your shoulders, hips, and feet should make a diagonal but straight line throughout this exercise. As you raise and lower your hips, brace your core, and engage your glutes to maximize your workout results.

Repeat this move for the assigned number of repetitions before switching to the other side. You should feel a strong burn throughout the side of your body, all the way through your glutes and shoulders. Never be afraid to take this one slower or at your own pace; after all, Side Plank Hip Dips can be as tricky to do as they are to say.

Form Tips

Practice this form in front of the mirror or a camera so that you can correctly assess how you are doing, and which areas need improvement. Be aware of where your elbow placement is underneath you. Ensure that your elbow stays directly under your shoulder, which will minimize any strain and help your back support your weight. Keep your head up and your shoulder away from your ears.

Make sure your body doesn't collapse forward and that your chest doesn't rotate towards the ground. Avoid this by keeping your core and glutes engaged, creating balance on both sides of your body.

Squat Pulses

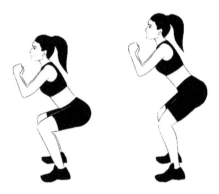

Squat Pulses are a very versatile version of the Squat exercise. Squat Pulses target all your glute muscles as well as your quads, hamstrings, and core muscles. You must execute this exercise as accurately as possible, or you face the possibility of spine- or waist-strain.

Instructions

Start by standing with your feet shoulder-width apart and your arms straight out in front of you, keeping your hands clasped together. Keep your back flat with your torso bent at a 45-degree angle. Make sure that your shoulders are back and that your core is braced. Tilt your pelvis forward as you lower your body as low as you can go until your thighs are parallel to the floor. You should feel your booty and hamstrings engage but maintain proper form and stop when you feel yourself overexerting. There are no added benefits the closer to the ground you get. If you go past the point of muscle engagement, the exercise isn't effective anymore, and your pelvis ends up taking on the strain.

Pulse a few inches, slightly lifting yourself up and dipping back down. This exercise is time-based rather than rep-based, so keep going until your time is up. You should be continuously squatting while keeping your knees bent to get that extra burn. You should try not to come back up to a standing position until your reps are completed. Be mindful of maintaining steady and purposeful breathing as you perform this exercise.

Form Tips

You must be wary of your knees and your back when doing Squat Pulses. Make sure your knees face outwards, giving you a lot of space for movement as you pulse up and down. Be aware of your knees passing too far over your toes, which is a sign that you are either curving your back or putting your weight into your toes instead of your heels.

If you notice that your form is off in this exercise, don't be afraid to stop and reset. Your ability to perform squat pulses over longer periods will increase as you get stronger and build up your stamina.

You must shake out your legs when finished with your Squat Pulses. If your lower body isn't used to this sort of movement, you may want to provide a little extra TLC to your muscles. You can also modify this exercise by not squatting as deep. What matters here is that your heels stay planted and that you're able to pulse a few inches while maintaining your form.

WEEK 1 WORKOUT PLAN

Over the next seven days, you'll have the opportunity to increase your reps gradually. Make sure you're doing an even number of repetitions per side. If the directions say to do 12 reps, you should do six on each side. Be sure to finish all the reps for one side before starting on the other!

Day 1

Day 1 Warm-Up

Begin your workout with the stretches and warm-ups of your choice from the ones we discussed. We're going to be executing a total of 12 reps per exercise for your workout today. If an exercise requires you to switch sides, you will be doing half of the reps on each side. For today, this means we'll be switching sides after 6 out of 12 total reps.

Clamshells

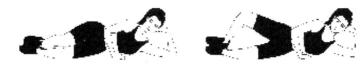

Donkey Kicks

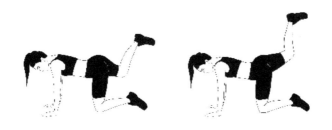

Day 1 Workout

Follow your warm-up with three rounds of the entire workout. This means doing each exercise and taking a quick breather before going through all of them two more times. Remember to practice purposeful breathing—take big, deep breaths as you slowly inhale and exhale. Don't forget to stretch and cool down when finishing your workout for the day! You've got this!

Glute Bridges (12 reps)

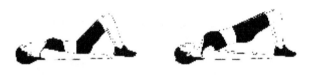

Straight Leg Hold (30 seconds per side)

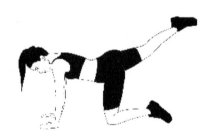

Side Plank Hip Dips (12 reps; 6 on each side)

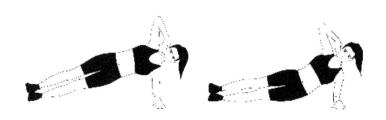

Day 2

Day 2 Warm-Up

Start your workout with the stretches and warm-ups of your choice. We're going to ramp things up today by doing a total of 14 repetitions. If the specific exercise you are doing requires you to switch sides, this means you'll be doing 7 of the 14 reps on each side.

Clamshells

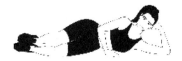 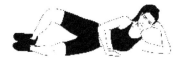

Dirty Dog

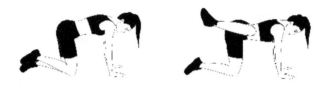

Day 2 Workout

Follow your warm-up with three rounds of the full workout. Don't forget to take a quick breather between sessions! After you are done with your three sets, don't forget to stretch and cool down before finishing your workout for the day! You're rocking it!

Single Leg Glute Bridge (14 reps; 7 on each side)

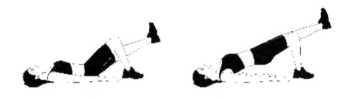

Straight Side Lift (14 reps; 7 on each side)

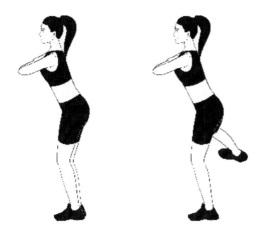

Squat Pulses (30 seconds)

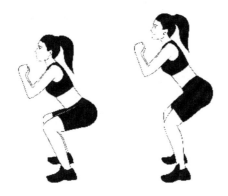

Day 3

Day 3 Warm-Up

As always, start your workout with the stretches and warm-ups of your choice. You've been doing such a great job that today; we're kicking it up another step! Your workout for today consists of a total of 16 repetitions per exercise! Don't forget to switch sides halfway through once you hit 8 of your 16 total reps.

Dirty Dog

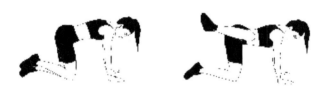

Donkey Kicks

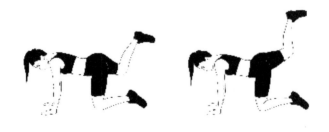

Day 3 Workout

After your warm-up, we will be doing three complete sets. Listen to your body when it tells you that you're pushing too hard. Practice your mindful breathing and take breaks between rounds. Don't forget to stretch afterward! You're doing fantastic work!

Glute Bridge (16 reps)

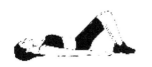 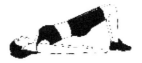

Outer Thigh Lift (16 reps; 8 on each side)

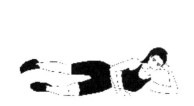 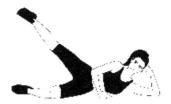

Side Plank Hip Dips (16 reps; 8 on each side)

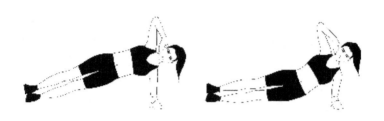

Day 4

Day 4 Warm-Up

Don't forget that you can always switch up your stretches and warm-ups. The important thing is to listen to your body. You've been doing such a great job that we're going to steady things out a little bit today by repeating yesterday's total of 16 repetitions. We'll be switching sides after 8 of the 16 total reps for the double-sided exercises.

Clamshells

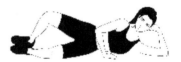

Donkey Kicks

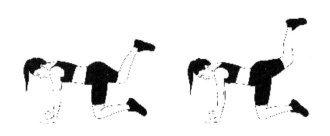

Day 4 Workout

By now, you should be getting used to completing three rounds of the whole workout. Remember to rest between sets and practice your breathing. It's essential to continue to stretch after your workouts, even if you are getting more used to them. Keep it up!

Single Leg Glute Bridge (16 reps; 8 on each side)

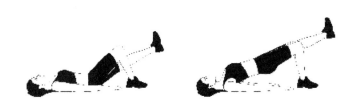

Straight Side Lift (45 seconds)

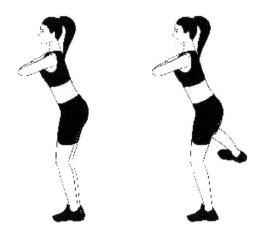

Squat Pulses (45 seconds)

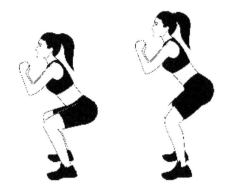

Day 5

Day 5 Warm-Up

Begin your workout with the stretches and warm-ups of your choice. We are going to go ahead and take things up another notch. That's right—we're going to complete 18 total reps for your workout today! Remember to switch sides halfway through when the exercise requires it. For today, that is after 9 out of your 18 repetitions are done.

Clamshell

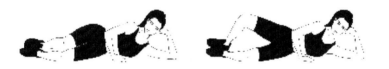

Dirty Dog

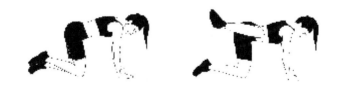

Day 5 Workout

Remember to follow your warm-up with three complete rounds of the workout. Be sure that you are listening to your body and not straining yourself. Take a quick breather between sets and take the time to stretch properly and cool down afterward. You're a workout queen!

Straight Leg Hold (30 seconds per side)

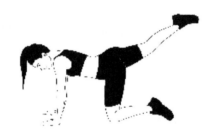

Outer Thigh Lifts (18 reps; 9 on each side)

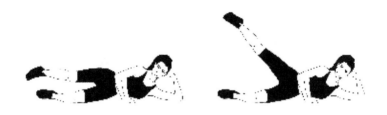

Side Plank Hip Dips (18 reps; 9 on each side)

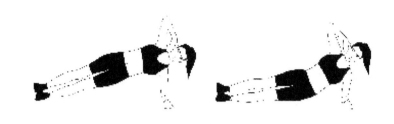

Day 6

Day 6 Warm-Up

Start off with your personal favorite stretches and warm-ups. We're going to turn the dial up on you again by executing 20 repetitions today! Of course, doing 20 repetitions means we'll be switching sides after 10 reps when the exercises require.

Dirty Dog

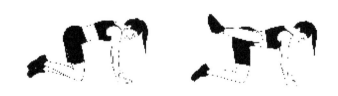

Donkey Kicks

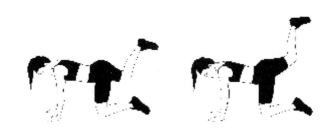

Day 6 Workout

You should still be doing three rounds of the total workout. Don't forget to take necessary rest breaks between sets, be mindful of your breathing, and stretch after you are done with your exercises. You've already come so far!

Glute Bridge (20 reps)

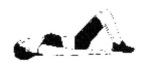 

Straight Side Lift (20 reps; 10 on each side)

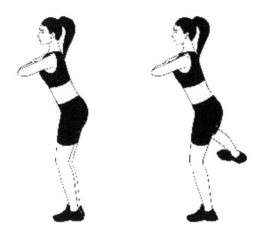

Squat Pulses (60 seconds)

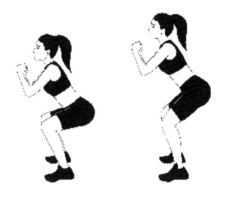

Day 7

Day 7 Warm-Up

Now that you've had plenty of practice using different stretches and activation exercises, which are your favorites? Make sure to begin your workout with those stretches and warm-ups! We're going to steady out a bit by executing another total of 20 reps per exercise, which means we'll be switching sides after every 10 out of 20 reps.

Clamshell

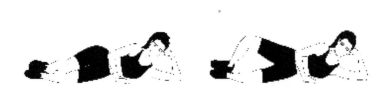

Donkey Kicks

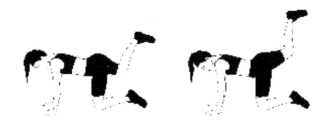

Day 7 Workout

Consistency is key, and now you are rocking out these three rounds! Remember how you balked at the idea of doing three whole sets when you first started just a week ago? Time sure flies! Remember to listen to your body, practice your breathing, and take rest breaks between sets. The next thing you know, you will be finishing your cool-down stretches, and your first week of workouts will be done!

Straight Leg Hold (60 seconds on each side)

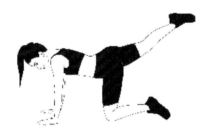

Single Leg Glute Bridge (20 reps; 10 on each side)

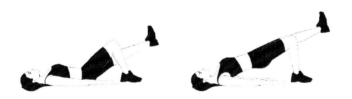

Outer Thigh Lift (20 reps; 10 on each side)

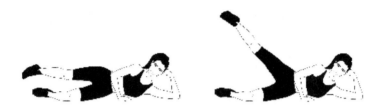

Congratulations! You completed your first week of the 14-Day Breakneck Booty Challenge! Pat yourself on the back and celebrate this outstanding achievement! But don't get too comfortable just yet—get ready to kick your butt into high gear by getting started on week two.

6

14 DAYS TO A BREAKNECK BOOTY: WEEK 2

You made it to the second week of your 14-Day Breakneck Booty Challenge! What an amazing accomplishment! You've come so far. You have much higher stamina, a firmer grasp of which stretches are your favorites, and so much more discipline. I hope you're feeling stronger and super proud of yourself. Give yourself a huge round of applause—you earned it!

Whether you're working out in the morning before your kids wake up, on your lunch break from work, or during your last few quiet hours before bed, you deserve to celebrate all of your hard work. You've taken the first huge step in your fitness journey. Just getting up and making yourself do the work is half the battle, but so many people don't even make it that far. You are proving that working out and looking after yourself can fit into any lifestyle.

Here comes the next step in your fitness journey: we're about to turn this challenge up! Now that you better understand the basics of fitness and your glutes, you're ready to push yourself a little bit further. This week, you'll be completing 20 to 30 repetitions of each move. But don't worry, you'll still be taking a one- to two-minute rest between each move. As this week gets more challenging, you might find yourself naturally needing more rest time or wanting to take more breaks. Your decision on the amount of rest time you need should be based on how you're feeling. It is better to take shorter breaks more frequently than to take fewer, longer ones. You want to keep your rest periods short to keep your heart rate up and your muscles engaged.

As you get into a routine and build up your stamina, try to mix things up a little bit this week. Taking shorter breaks is an excellent way to challenge yourself more, but don't overexert yourself! Try to reach a deeper squat, hold a pose, or stretch longer, and engage your abs more. Only you know what your body is capable of and how far you can push yourself! Always remember to take five or ten minutes to stretch out your muscles and get your blood moving. Stretch both before and after your workout. Refer to Chapter 3 if you need to review your stretches; don't forget that you can pick-and-choose stretches based on how you're feeling each day.

WEEK 2 EXERCISES

Let's start by breaking down the exercises you'll be executing this week. Be sure to read over the descriptions thoroughly and practice your form before starting your workout. Being careful while learning the movements benefits you in the long run by setting you up to avoid injury and strain.

Your exercises for this week are High Bridge Pulses, Side Lift Pulses, Straight Leg Pulses, Spider Plank Crunches, Forward Leaning Split Squats, Outer Thigh Circles, Hamstring Curls, Standing Kickbacks, and Single Leg Deadlifts.

High Bridge Pulses

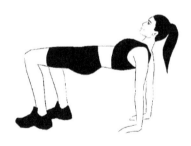

Now that you've learned how to execute the Glute Bridge and the Single Leg Glute Bridge, it's time to level up. The High Bridge Pulse targets your gluteus maximus, lower back, hamstrings, and calves. High Bridge Pulses are great for maximizing your benefits by working out your entire lower body.

Instructions

This exercise is very similar to the Glute Bridge, but this variation adds intensity by also engaging your upper body. Begin by lying on your back with your feet shoulder-width apart and with your knees bent, pointing upward. Place your hands palm-side down with your fingers pointing towards your feet. Make sure your shoulders are touching the mat or the floor beneath you.

Using your arms, push yourself up into a high bridge position. Keep your spine flat, your knees bent at a 90-degree angle, and your arms straight. Lower your hips as you did in the earlier bridge exercises, keeping your arms extended. Once your knees are at about a 45-degree angle, pulse your hips back up so that your knees, hips, and shoulders form a horizontal line. Squeeze your glutes at the top of the movement, keeping your core engaged. Be sure that you keep your core engaged to prevent overextending your back.

After completing your reps, return your hips down flat to the ground, and reset. You should feel a massive burn throughout your glutes as you execute this exercise and as you rest following it. Your back should be free of pain, however. If you're feeling any strain in your back, double-check that you're putting the work into your glutes and using your arms and core to stabilize yourself.

Form Tips

You must keep your spine neutral and flat by drawing your hips and pushing your shoulders down. Don't release tension and relax at the lowest point of your pulse. Instead, keep the tension during the entire movement by squeezing even more at the height of the motion. If you're unsure of your form, watch yourself in the mirror or take a video of yourself to check.

Side Lift Pulses

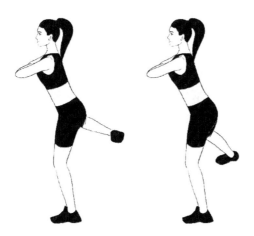

Side Lift Pulses easily adapt to your everyday lifestyle. You can practice Side Lift Pulses anywhere that you can stand, even while you're watching TV. This exercise targets your gluteus medius and your gluteus minimus. Get ready to feel that burn!

Instructions

Just like in the Straight Side Lift, stand up and balance on your right foot with your hands in front of you. If balancing is too difficult, try holding onto a wall or chair for stability. Instead of raising your straight leg, bend your knee at a 90-degree angle.

As you raise your leg, keep your knee bent and feel for the stretch in your upper booty. When you reach the top of the motion, bring your knee halfway back to your other leg. Pulse back up to the top of the motion. Your bent leg should remain tense and lifted for the entire movement.

Form Tips

Avoid bringing your leg too high when pulsing, as you could shift your hips off-center or overextend your back. You shouldn't feel any pressure in your lower back for the duration of this exercise.

As your muscles get tired, you might find it easier to throw your leg up and let it drop. Not only is relying on momentum dangerous and can lead to injury, but it also takes away any actual work from your muscles or benefits from your workout. Remember the importance of practicing proper breathing techniques, maintaining your form, and using your muscles rather than momentum to perform the exercise.

Straight Leg Pulses

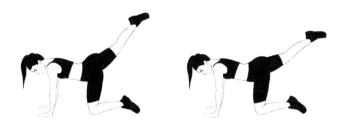

Straight Leg Pulses are a winning combo of Side Lift Pulses and the Straight Leg Hold. Straight Leg Pulses engage your core as well as your glutes. Trust yourself, trust your balance, and trust all the work you've done so far.

Instructions

Get into the same starting Tabletop Pose as the Straight Leg Hold and extend one leg straight back behind you with a flexed foot. From here, raise your leg upwards until you feel your glutes engage. Be sure to squeeze at the top before pulsing your way back down. Go up and down like this for each rep, keeping these muscles engaged and tense through the entire movement.

Form Tips

For this exercise, pay particular attention to your core to avoid overextending and straining your back. Keep your gaze forward and moving with your body, rather than straining to stare in one spot. If you look straight ahead, you can avoid straining your neck.

Spider Plank Crunch

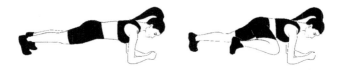

The Spider Plank Crunch serves as an advanced crunch form. It targets your core, obliques, and hip flexors as well as your triceps, so get ready to feel the burn! This exercise can be tricky and can present some strain on your neck when executed incorrectly, so go through this workout slowly at first until you feel confident that you are moving correctly.

Instructions

Start in a Plank Pose with your shoulders, hips, and knees in a straight line, with your wrists directly under your shoulders. Bend one knee outwards and pull it in towards the corresponding shoulder in a crunch-like motion. Then return to the Plank Pose and repeat on the other side.

You want to look like Spider-Man climbing up the side of a building. Keep your core and glutes engaged as you imagine you are a superhero for a few reps. Sometimes pretending to be a superhero or a supervillain can take your mind off the burn you're feeling; it refocuses your energy into the fun and joy that comes with exercise. This is your time—play around, make it the best time it can be for you!

Form Tips

Keep your abs and glutes tense to prevent your hips from sinking, straining your back, or generally injuring yourself. Keep your neck in a neutral position and your eyes looking directly down. Do not lower your head to look under yourself or at your legs, and do not twist your head up to look at the wall. Both of those awkward movements could lead to neck strain and injury.

Be sure to tighten your core and obliques as you pull in your knees to create stability. This movement will ensure you're targeting the right muscles. When we don't engage our muscles, we throw our form off or target the wrong muscles, thus leading to strain or injury.

Forward Leaning Split Squat

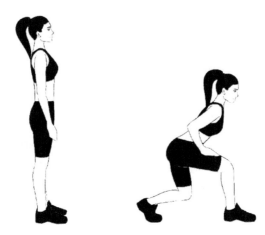

The Forward Leaning Split Squat is great for your flexibility and leg strength since it helps to tone your lower booty and keep your knees limber. The mobility of your knees and hips is important, so exercises like this will significantly help your fitness journey, especially when you're working out without a lot of time. You want compound moves that target more muscles and engage the most parts of your body at once to achieve those killer results in less time.

The Forward Leaning Split Squat engages the gluteus maximus muscles, as well as your hip flexors, hamstrings, and abductors. This exercise is the real deal—it's a complete lower-body move.

Instructions

Stand in a lunge stance with one foot in front of your body and the other foot behind you, but with both feet still shoulder-width apart. Engage your core by placing your hands on your hips for the duration of this exercise. If you were to start on your right leg, your right heel should be two to four feet in front of your left foot; raise your left heel to evenly distribute your weight on your toes.

Begin the downward movement by bending your right leg's hip, knee, and ankle while lowering your left knee to the ground. Lean forward with your upper body and keep your upper body over your right knee. Leaning forward helps to target that outer hip and to get your booty working over-time. Lower your body until your right leg is parallel to the floor, with your left knee underneath your rear hip, hovering about one to two inches off the ground.

Hold the squat for a few seconds, then use the weight in your right foot to engage and push yourself upwards. Keep your chest high and open while squeezing your front glute as you stand.

Form Tips

Always be aware of your neck movements, and keep your chin tucked throughout the entire movement. Keep an eye on where your front knee is as you squat. Ensure it stays behind your toes to avoid overextension of your back leg and unnecessary pressure on your knee joint. Make sure your back leg stays at a 90-degree angle as you squat. If you do this squat with a straight back leg, you stress your hip joints, knee joint, and surrounding muscles.

Outer Thigh Circles

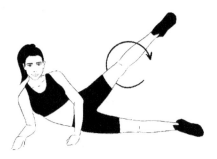

Outer Thigh Circles are an excellent exercise to strengthen your hip joints and hamstrings. This move helps lubricate your joints and builds your range of motion. Outer Thigh Circles work your abductors, gluteus maximus, gluteus medius, and gluteus minimus, which means you are getting an entire booty workout!

Instructions

Lie down on your right side and bend your right bottom arm to support your head. Your left hand should be resting on the floor directly in front of you for stability. You should extend your right bottom leg straight below you as you lie flat on the floor.

Flex your left foot and raise your left leg, slowly moving it in a circular motion. Do the assigned number of repetitions in a clockwise motion, then repeat them going counterclockwise before switching legs. If this feels a little too advanced for you, just make your circles a little smaller.

Form Tips

As you move your top leg, you might notice your hips and core moving around a bit. Be sure to engage and pull in your abs and glutes to create a firm base for yourself. Make sure that your pelvis stays stable as you rotate your leg.

Hamstring Curl

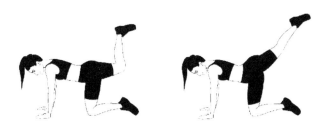

Hamstring Curls are a crucial exercise to incorporate into your workouts. The hamstring is a huge muscle that requires a lot of training to achieve its peak ability—it helps you run, jog, jump, deadlift, and squat. The hamstring is an easily injured muscle, your form is really important here; otherwise, you may find yourself out of commission for a while. This exercise targets your hamstrings as well as your quadriceps and your glutes. Hamstring Curls are an entire lower-body exercise, and they may even aid you with balance training!

Instructions

Stand upright with your feet hip-width apart, placing your hands on your hips or a chair for balance. From standing, shift your weight to your left leg. Slowly bend your right knee, bringing your heel up toward your butt while keeping your thighs parallel. For an extra burn, hold for a few seconds at the top of the movement. Slowly lower your foot to the starting position. Repeat this exercise for the assigned number of repetitions before switching sides. You can also do this exercise on all fours with your right leg extended behind you.

Form Tips

Engage your abs during this exercise to avoid arching your back. Your legs should be the only thing bending during this move. Move slowly and with control. Make sure to squeeze your hamstring muscle when you fully curl.

Standing Kickbacks

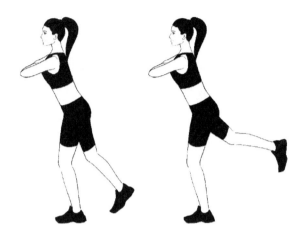

Standing Kickbacks can be difficult for balancing, but they target so many different muscles. Your body will thank you. Standing Kickbacks target your gluteus maximus, legs, and abs when executed correctly.

Instructions

Stand upright with your arms out in front of you and your right leg slightly behind your left leg. If you need assistance with balance, feel free to place your hands on your hips or hold onto a chair for support. Although you can start off using an object for support and balance, we want to work up to relying on your core for stability as you get more used to the movement. Mastering your balance takes time, so listen to your body and trust your work.

Slowly extend your right leg behind you for as far as you can without arching your back. Don't forget to engage and contract your core and glute muscles. Pause at the top of the motion and hold your form for a few seconds before lowering your leg and returning to your starting position. Finish all of the repetitions on one side before repeating them on the opposite side. Be sure to keep the number of repetitions even on each side.

Form Tips

Practicing your balance will help you succeed in this exercise. Be sure to keep your abs engaged at all times and your glutes engaged as you pull your leg up. Bending your knee slightly, rather than locking it up, also helps with avoiding injury or strain.

Be aware of your back and make sure you aren't arching it in order to avoid back injury. Keeping your back straight also ensures that you are keeping your work in the right muscle groups.

Single Leg Deadlift

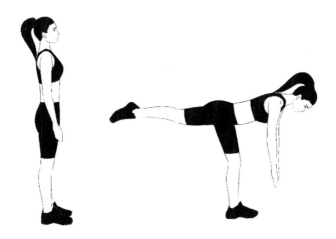

The Single Leg Deadlift relies on a lot of balance, core work, and glute action. Single Leg Deadlifts are one of those exercises that you can always find ways to improve and add onto for more of a challenge. Keep this exercise in your back pocket as you move forward. Single Leg Deadlifts target your leg muscles, hip mobility, glutes, and core to create a well-rounded lower body.

Instructions

Start with your feet hip-width apart underneath you, placing your left arm on your hip while the right is at your side. Ensure that your whole body is stacked from your ankles to your shoulders and that your spine stays neutral. Engage your core as you step your left leg back slightly and begin to hinge your hips.

Lift your left leg straight and up behind you, lowering your torso until it is parallel to the floor. Create a straight line from your head to your toes. Your glutes and core must stay engaged in this position. Reach your right arm that was at your side down towards the floor for support. Pause and hold for a few seconds at the top of the motion, then put your weight into your right heel as you slowly lower your left foot back down to the ground. Bring your torso upright once again to return to the starting position.

Form Tips

Single Leg Deadlifts are extremely challenging. Keep your back straight during the hinge forward. Be aware of where you are looking to help keep your neck as neutral as possible.

Be aware of your right arm when you reach down. You do not necessarily need to touch the floor, especially if doing so means sacrificing your form through your spine. Use your arm as a kickstand to help with balance if you need to, but it is not necessary to touch the ground in this exercise.

WEEK 2 WORKOUT PLAN

Are you ready for the second week of your 14-day challenge? You already conquered the first week, so this week should be a breeze. Get ready to level up, challenge yourself, and work your booty. You'll be starting your week at 22 repetitions, but by the end of the challenge, you'll be flying through 30 reps of each exercise. It's going to be a challenge—remember to breathe correctly and listen to your body. This workout is for you and your benefit, so pay attention to how you feel each day. You got this!

Day 8

Day 8 Warm-Up

Begin your workout with the stretches and warm-ups of your choice. Refer back to Chapter 3 for some of the different stretches you can try. For an added challenge, try a stretch you didn't use last week. We will execute a total of 22 reps for your workout today; this means we'll be switching sides after 11 reps when necessary.

Clamshells

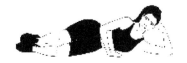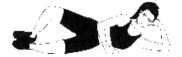

Donkey Kicks

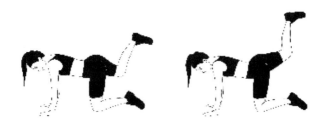

Day 8 Workout

It's time for your full workout! You may notice that we are now doing four base exercises rather than three. However, we're still going to do a total of three rounds of your four exercises today. It is perfectly acceptable to take a breather or short rest between each round. Please also remember to stretch and cool down when you are finished with the main exercises. You are doing fantastic work so far—keep it up!

Straight Leg Pulses (60 seconds; 30 seconds per side)

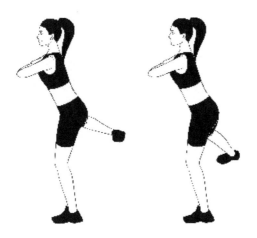

High Bridge Pulse (30 seconds)

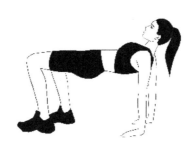

Forward Leaning Split Squat (22 reps; 11 on each side)

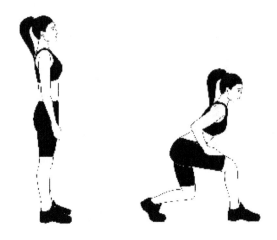

Single Leg Deadlift (22 reps; 11 on each side)

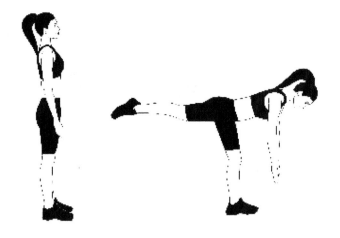

Day 9

Day 9 Warm-Up

Don't forget to take the time to stretch and warm up first. Pick the warm-up stretches that make you feel the most limber and ready. Today, we're going to execute 22 reps of each exercise. Be sure to switch sides halfway through your repetitions when doing a double-sided exercise.

Clamshells

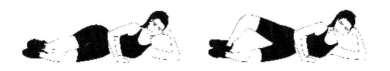

Dirty Dog

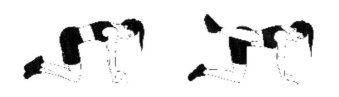

Day 9 Workout

We will continue to do three rounds of these four different exercises. Remember to take each round at your own pace and listen to your body. Keep practicing proper breathing techniques throughout. Take a short break between rounds and start from the top again. As always, stretch afterward as part of your cool down.

Spider Plank Crunch (22 reps; 11 on each side)

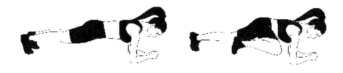

Side Lift Pulses (22 reps; 11 on each side)

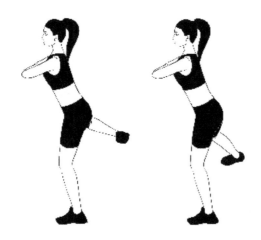

Outer Thigh Circles (22 reps; 11 on each side)

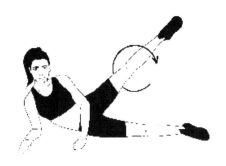

Single Leg Deadlift (22 reps; 11 on each side)

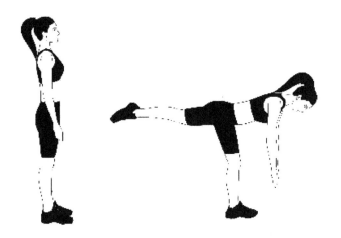

Day 10

Day 10 Warm-Up

Begin with the stretches of your choice before starting your activation exercises. We will bump up our total number of repetitions to 24 reps of each exercise today, meaning that the halfway mark to switch sides is at 12 reps.

Dirty Dog

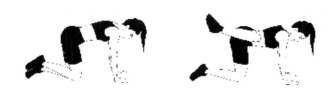

Donkey Kicks

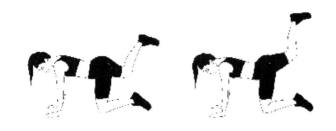

Day 10 Workout

Even though we are doing four different exercises, continue doing three whole rounds for a full workout. Be sure to take water breaks and rest between each round as needed. Maintain proper breathing and form; this means moving slowly, steadily, and purposefully to avoid straining yourself. When you are done with your three rounds, remember to stretch again afterward.

Hamstring Curl (24 reps; 12 on each side)

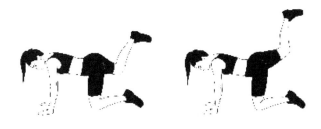

Forward Leaning Split Squat (24 reps; 12 on each side)

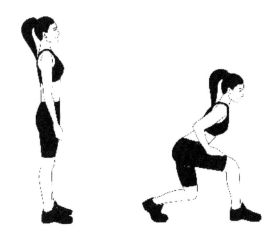

Bridge Pulse (30 seconds)

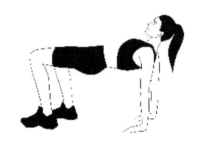

Single Leg Deadlift (24 reps; 12 on each side)

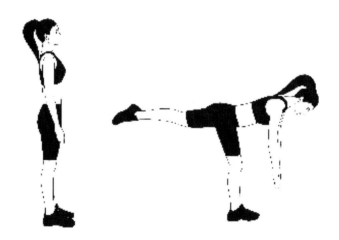

Day 11

Day 11 Warm-Up

Look at you! You're already halfway through your second week! Let your progress invigorate you to keep going! Begin today with the stretches of your choice. We will steady out a bit and keep our repetitions at 24 for today, switching halfway at 12 reps when necessary.

Clamshells

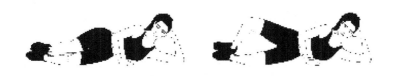

Donkey Kick

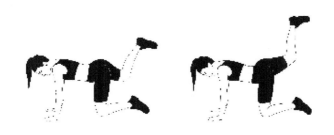

Day 11 Workout

Once you complete your warm-up, execute three rounds of your total workout. Keep some water close by so that you stay hydrated. It's okay to take short water breaks between rounds as you need them. Be careful not to strain yourself by being mindful of your breathing techniques and form. Stretching afterward also helps avoid possible strain or injury. Believe in yourself—you're doing exceptional work!

Straight leg pulses (24 reps; 12 on each side)

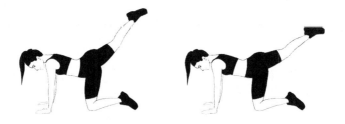

Outer Thigh Circles (24 reps; 12 on each side)

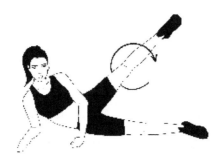

Kickbacks (24 reps; 12 on each side)

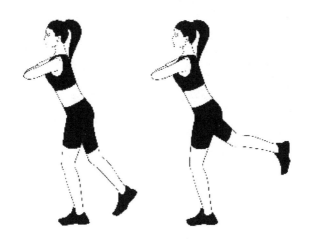

Single Leg Deadlift (24; 12 on each side)

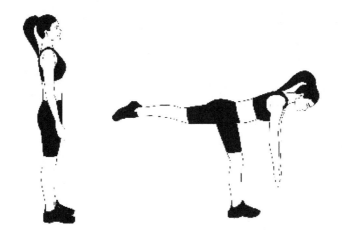

Day 12

Day 12 Warm-Up

It's time to kick things up another notch! Today, we're following our stretches up with 26 repetitions! Switch sides halfway through your repetitions, which means you are doing 13 reps for each side today. Listen to your body by resting between breaks when you need to and staying hydrated.

Clamshells

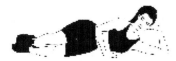 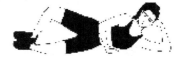

Dirty Dog

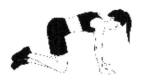 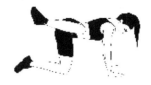

Day 12 Workout

You're so close to the end now! Don't give up! Pay attention to your form today. As your muscles fatigue throughout these two weeks, you might begin to lose your form. Take the time to ensure your body is aligned correctly and that you're executing each exercise safely and properly. Enjoy feeling the strength and control of your muscles performing the movements rather than letting momentum do them for you. Leave time for you to complete your stretches afterward.

Spider Plank Crunch (26 reps; 13 on each side)

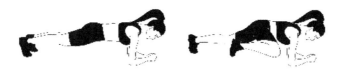

Hamstring Curl (26 reps; 13 on each side)

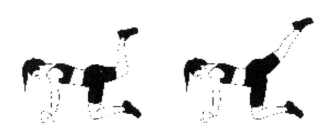

Forward Leaning Split Squat (26 reps; 13 on each side)

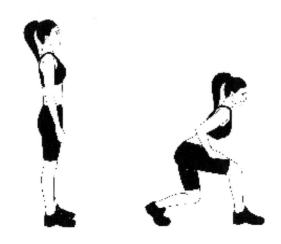

Single Leg Deadlift (26 reps; 13 on each side)

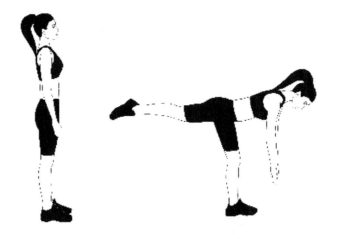

Day 13

Day 13 Warm-Up

Start off with your stretches, and try to stretch a little deeper today. How are your muscles feeling? Try to utilize stretches that address and relieve the muscles that are the sorest. We're going to bring our number of total repetitions up to 28 today, which means switching sides at 14 reps for double-sided exercises.

Dirty Dog

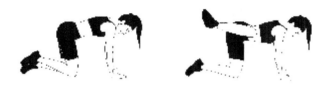

Donkey Kicks

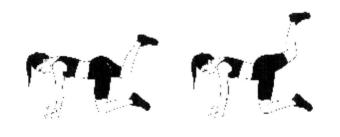

Day 13 Workout

Remember to do three whole rounds of the set of four exercises for a complete workout. Practice your purposeful breathing and controlled movement. Pace yourself by taking breaks between rounds but leave yourself enough time to stretch when you are finished. You got this!

Straight leg pulses (28 reps; 14 on each side)

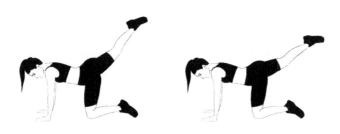

High Bridge Pulses (60 seconds)

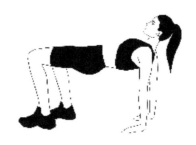

Kickbacks (28 reps; 14 on each side)

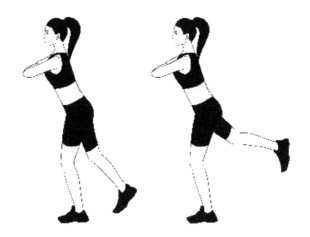

Single Leg Deadlift (28 reps; 14 on each side)

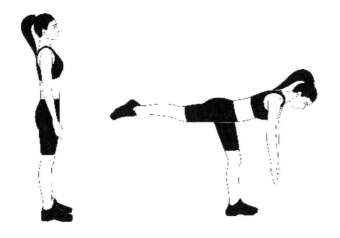

Day 14

Day 14 Warm-Up

Today is the last day of your challenge, so really give it all you've got! You can see the finish line! Begin with the stretches of your choice before starting your activation exercises. We're doing 30 repetitions of each movement, switching sides halfway through when you hit 15 repetitions.

Clamshells

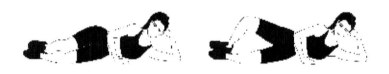

Donkey Kicks

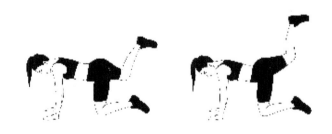

Day 14 Workout

It's the moment you've been waiting for: it's time for your final three rounds! If you feel overwhelmed, take it five minutes at a time. You can do anything for five minutes. Believe in your body and the strength you've built over the past two weeks. Remember to practice steady breathing, proper form techniques, and stretching when you finish. You're a powerhouse! Listen to your body and have fun!

Spider Plank Crunches (30 reps; 15 on each side)

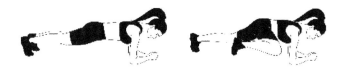

Side Lift Pulses (30 reps; 15 on each side)

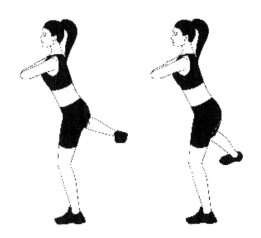

Kickbacks (30 reps; 15 on each side)

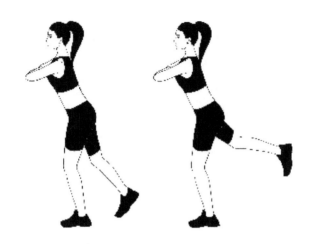

Single Leg Deadlift (30 reps; 15 on each side)

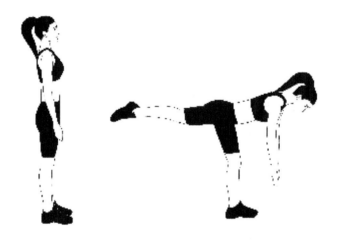

You did it! Way to go! That's two weeks of hard work in the bag!

How do you feel? Go get some water and reward yourself. You just completed a goal you set for yourself. You didn't give up! Maybe you wavered a bit and felt tested, but you didn't give up. Even with your time restraints and busy schedule, you persevered. What comes next is up to you. Be proud of all the work you've done in this challenge—I sure am!

CONCLUSION

Congratulations! You completed your 14-Day Breakneck Booty Challenge! What a major accomplishment! Go ahead and pat yourself on the back to celebrate. You've already taken the first major steps in creating a healthier and stronger you!

Your health and fitness are vital to ensuring that you have a long and capable life. You don't need to spend hours in the gym or hundreds of dollars on exercise equipment. Everything you need to reach your dream body is within your grasp.

No matter how busy you get, you've proven that you can do the hardest part: adding fitness into your everyday routine as part of your lifestyle. You can always find a few minutes for your fitness and wellbeing. Getting up and moving your body each day can be just as effective as a gym membership.

The power is within you. You spent the last 14 days strengthening your booty and your lower body, so don't stop now! You proved to yourself that working out for 14 consecutive days is possible. Remember, we want to make a breakneck body, not just a breakneck booty. After you complete your two-week challenge, I recommend working your glutes no more than three times a week so that you don't burn out. Leave time for your muscles to recoup and recover. Be sure to work out other muscle groups on your off days.

The choice to invest in your body is no one's but your own. You never need to feel unhappy or disappointed in how you look. You've found a quick and easy solution to your problem. The world is now your oyster. You have your baseline stretches, routine, and form down. You're ready to tackle anything and everything.

Now you know firsthand that any woman, no matter her lifestyle, can make time for her own fitness and health. You are a walking example of the strength that we working women have within us. You defy the restraints women are put under by proving that women can be strong, fit, and healthy while working and looking after their families. You don't need to sacrifice your own happiness and health for the nine-to-five lifestyle or a perfect family. You can and should have it all!

I'm honored to be a part of your fitness journey thus far. Your work and progress over the last two weeks have been amazing. Be proud of yourself, celebrate yourself, and get moving again tomorrow. Your journey is just getting started. I am always busy writing more books for you so that we can tackle every area of our body, so keep your eyes peeled. We don't just want a breakneck booty; we have our eyes on a breakneck body!

After your booty gets some recovery time, don't be afraid to do these 14-day exercises again and again. They'll always be here for you if you're ever looking for a quick and easy workout to kickstart your fitness. I'll always be here for you on your fitness journey, but I'll especially be available if you join our Breakneck Booty Squad on Facebook!

Go check out and join our Breakneck Body Squad on Facebook. The Breakneck Body Squad is a community I've created for all of us to share our progress, major wins, favorite exercises, workout videos, form and posture tips, and even healthy recipes! It is a positive, encouraging, and safe space to share, track, ask questions, motivate, and make connections with other women on their fitness adventures. I urge you to like, interact, and support each other over there. I will always be available inside the Breakneck Body Squad community to ensure your further success and to workout with you!

Thanks for joining me these past two weeks. I hope you recognize the incredible feat you accomplished. Always remember to thank your body. Look at yourself in the mirror and thank your body for helping you achieve this, holding you up, and growing with you. Thank your body for all it does for you. You may not have your dream body yet, but that doesn't mean your body isn't worthwhile. Your body is a beautiful temple that just got you through 14 days of hard work. Thank it the same way you'd thank someone for helping you achieve a personal life goal.

If you enjoyed this or learned something, please pass it along to your friends. Encourage your working female friends who are feeling stuck in that same rut to kick-start their journey with you. You completed your goal, so you are the example now! Go forth and be that example to other women like you.

All women deserve to feel strong and beautiful. All women deserve some 'me-time' to focus on themselves and look after themselves. All women deserve other women cheering them on and helping them become the best version of themselves they can be, no matter their age, job position, and marital or parental status. You are a strong woman who just completed a 14-day challenge. Celebrate and be proud. You are unstoppable!

REFERENCES

8fit Team. (n.d.). *How to do lunges correctly: a beginner's guide.* 8fit. https://8fit.com/fitness/lunges-right-beginners-guide/

Akram, M. (2021, April 1). *Bodyweight hamstring exercises to do at home.* TheFitnessPhantom. https://thefitnessphantom. com/bodyweight-hamstring-exercises/

Anjorin, K. (2020, Dec 16). *25 Best Butt Exercises For Super-Toned Glute Muscles.* Women's Health Magazine. https:// www.womenshealthmag.com/fitness/a19983280/best-butt-exercises/

Axe, C. (2017, June 22). *Gluteus maximus: The exercises, stretches, and injuries to avoid for your glutes!* Dr. Axe. https:// draxe.com/fitness/gluteus-maximus/

Braverman, J. (2019, June 13). *What are leg kickback exercises?* (A. Bailey, PT, DPT, CHT, Ed.). LIVESTRONG.COM. https://www.livestrong.com/article/411281-what-are-leg-kick-back-exercises/

Burgie, A. (2013). *Overcoming obstacles to get in shape.* Get Holistic Health. https://www.getholistichealth.com/29901/overcoming-obstacles-to-get-in-shape/

Chertoff, J. (2019, April 9). *Lunges: muscles worked, how-to, variations, and more* (D. Bubnis, Ed.). Healthline. https://www.healthline.com/health/fitness-exercise/lunges-muscles-worked#takeaway

Dale, P. (2020, June 12). *Split squat exercise guide: How-To, muscles worked, variations, and benefits.* Fitness Volt. https://fitnessvolt.com/split-squat/

De Medeiros, M. (2018, July 29.) *10 No-Equipment Moves for a Tighter, Toner Butt.* PopSugar. https://www.popsugar.com/fitness/photo-gallery/45000635/image/45000642/Standing-Kickbacks

ePainAssist. (2017, March 6). 5 *Exercises for outer thigh that strengthen and tone your legs.* EPainAssist. https://www.epainassist.com/fitness-and-exercise/5-exercises-for-outer-thigh-that-strengthen-and-tone-your-legs

Focus Fitness. (2019, July 12). *How to do spiderman plank crunch exercise properly.* Flab Fix. https://flabfix.com/how-to-do-plank-crunch-exercise-properly/

Holder, J. (2021, March 17). *How to do split squats with perfect form.* Masterclass. https://www.masterclass.com/articles/ split-squat-guide#want-to-dive-deeper-into-your-wellness-journey

How to do the glute bridge. (2013). *Glute bridge: How to do it, benefits and variations.* Coach. https://www.coachmag.co.uk/ glute-exercises/2333/glute-bridge-how-to-do-it-benefits-and-variations

Jolie. (2015, July 18). *Buttocks anatomy 101—glute muscles explained.* Betterbuttchallenge.com. https:// betterbuttchallenge.com/buttocks-anatomy-101-glute-muscles-explained/

Kanski, CPT, L. (2019, October 18). *How to do the fire hydrant exercise, according to a trainer.* Women's Health. https://www. womenshealthmag.com/fitness/a29392097/fire-hydrant-exercise/

Kester, S. (2019, July 24). *Side leg raises two ways with variations and tips.* Healthline. https://www.healthline.com/ health/side-leg-raises#about

Lefkowith, C. (2015, December 9). *Side plank hip dips.* Redefining Strength. https://redefiningstrength.com/side-plank-hip-dips/

Maguire, J. (2017, October 31). *Clamshell exercise: how and why you should do it.* Openfit. https://www.openfit.com/ clamshell-exercise

Maguire, J. (2018, May 11). *Side plank hip lifts exercise: How to do it properly.* Openfit. https://www.openfit.com/side-plank-hip-lifts

Mahaffey, K. (n.d.). *How to do a glute bridge: form, workouts, and more.* Blog.nasm.org. https://blog.nasm.org/how-to-do-a-glute-bridge

MasterClass Staff. (2021, April 26). *How to do single leg glute bridges with perfect form.* Masterclass.com. https://www.masterclass.com/articles/single-leg-glute-bridge-guide#what-is-a-singleleg-glute-bridge

Mayo Clinic Staff. (2019, May 11). *7 great reasons why exercise matters.* Mayo Clinic. https://www.mayoclinic.org/healthy-lifestyle/fitness/in-depth/exercise/art-20048389

Mayo Clinic Staff. (2019). *Barriers to fitness: Overcoming common challenges.* Mayo Clinic. https://www.mayoclinic.org/healthy-lifestyle/fitness/in-depth/fitness/art-20045099

Nunez, K. (2019, May 23). *Fire hydrant exercise: technique, benefits, and tips.* Healthline. https://www.healthline.com/health/exercise-fitness/fire-hydrant-exercise#modified-versions

Osnato, J. (2020, January 24). *5-minutes glute activation routine to always do before a butt workout.* Livestrong.com https://www.livestrong.com/article/13724260-glute-activation-exercises/

Quinn, E. (2020, September 1). *Do a single leg bridge exercise for butt and core.* Verywell Fit. https://www.verywellfit.com/single-leg-bridge-exercise-3120739

Schultz, R. (2019, May 10). *How to do a Single Leg Deadlift— benefits, form and workouts.* Women's Health Magazine. https://www.womenshealthmag.com/fitness/a27423100/single-leg-deadlift-exercise/

Spiderman Crunch. (n.d.). *Spiderman crunch form, muscles worked, benefits.* Homegym-Exercises.com. https://homegym-exercises.com/spiderman_crunch.html

Sprow, MPH, CSCS, K. (2019, August 2). *Paradigm shift in physical activity research: Do bouts matter?* ACSM.org. https://www.acsm.org/all-blog-posts/acsm-blog/acsm-blog/2019/08/02/physical-activity-research-bouts-duration

The Pilates Studio. (2013, April 14). *Exercise of the day: Day 288—side lying leg circles up and over the magic circle.* The Pilates Studio. http://pilatesexerciseoftheday.blogspot.com/2013/04/day-288-side-lying-leg-circles-up-and.html

Thomason, K., & Sullivan, CPT, J. (2019, April 12). *How to do a donkey kick to strengthen your glutes.* Women's Health. https://www.womenshealthmag.com/fitness/a27115760/donkey-kicks/

UW Health. (2017, March 21). *Is 20 minutes of exercise enough?* www.uwhealth.org. https://www.uwhealth.org/news/is-20-minutes-of-exercise-enough

Vorvick, MD., L. J. (2019, May 13). *Sacrum.* Medlineplus.gov. https://medlineplus.gov/ency/imagepages/19464. htm#:~:text=The%20sacrum%20is%20a%20shield

Webb, M. (2011, September 8). *Increase energy levels and cure fatigue through exercise.* Acefitness.org. https://www. acefitness.org/education-and-resources/lifestyle/blog/ 6589/increase-energy-levels-and-cure-fatigue-through- exercise/

Weir, J. (2019, June 13). *What muscles do side leg raises work?* LIVESTRONG.COM. https://www.livestrong.com/article/ 539306-what-muscles-do-side-leg-raises-work/

Wolfe, L. M. (n.d.). *How to do the outer thigh raise exercise.* Live Healthy - Chron.com. https://livehealthy.chron.com/outer- thigh-raise-exercise-6442.html

Zeller, V. (Ed.). (n.d.). *Standing glute kickback: How to do guide, modifications, pro tips and videos.* Fitstop24.com. https:// fitstop24.com/exercise/standing-glute-kickback/